Plants in cosmetics

**Plants and plant preparations
used as ingredients
for cosmetic products
Volume II**

prepared by the Committee of Experts on Cosmetic Products
with the collaboration of

Prof. Robert Anton, consultant (France)
Dr Franco Patri, consultant (Italy)
Prof. Vittorio Silano, consultant (Italy)

Les plantes
dans les cosmétiques

**Plantes et préparations
à base de plantes utilisées
en tant qu'ingrédients
dans les produits cosmétiques
Volume II**

élaboré par le Comité d'experts sur les produits cosmétiques
avec la collaboration de

Prof. Robert Anton, consultant (France)
Dr Franco Patri, consultant (Italie)
Prof. Vittorio Silano, consultant (Italie)

Health protection of the consumer
Protection de la santé du consommateur

Council of Europe Publishing
Editions du Conseil de l'Europe

Cover design and layout: Pre-press Unit of the Council of Europe
Edited by the Partial Agreement Department in the Social and Public Health Field and Council of Europe Publishing

http://book.coe.int

Council of Europe Publishing
F-67075 Strasbourg Cedex

ISBN 92-871-4676-4
© Council of Europe, September 2001
Printed in Germany by Koelblin-Fortuna-Druck

Contents/Sommaire

Preamble

Fields of activity of the Council of Europe

The competence of the Council of Europe is very wide and covers practically all aspects of European affairs, with the exception of defence matters. Where, however, a lesser number of states wish to engage in some action in which not all their European partners desire to join, they can conclude a "partial agreement" which is binding on themselves alone.

Partial Agreement in the Social and Public Health Field

It was on this basis that the Partial Agreement in the Social and Public Health Field was concluded in 1959 by the Council of Europe Committee of Ministers and revised in 1996 by the Committee of Ministers with effect from 1 January 1997. The following states are Members of the Partial Agreement: Austria, Belgium, Cyprus, Denmark, Finland, France, Germany, Ireland, Italy, Luxembourg, the Netherlands, Norway, Portugal, Spain, Sweden, Switzerland and the United Kingdom of Great Britain and Northern Ireland.

The aim of the Partial Agreement public health activities is to protect the consumer from potential risks connected with the present-day way of life. The Committees of Experts provide the scientific base for national and international regulations concerning products which have a direct or indirect impact on the human food chain (control of foodstuffs, nutrition, food safety, consumer health, food contact materials, flavouring substances), pesticides, pharmaceuticals and cosmetics.

The Steering Committee responsible for the activities concerning health protection of the consumer is the Public Health Committee, composed of high-ranking Ministry of Health officials of the member states. It supervises the Committees of Experts' activities and specifies the general principles of the public health policy which these Committees have to follow in their work.

The Partial Agreement in the Social and Public Health Field has always closely followed technical evolution and scientific progress and resolutions, guidelines and reports arising from its work are often of a pioneering nature.

In most fields, the approach is that of toxicological evaluation of chemical substance groups, the setting of technical and toxicological specifications, elaboration of maximum or guideline levels and preparation of inventory lists of chemical substances used by industry.

Avant-propos

Domaines d'activité du Conseil de l'Europe

La compétence du Conseil de l'Europe est très large et englobe pratiquement tous les aspects des affaires européennes, à l'exception des questions de défense. Si, toutefois, un certain nombre d'Etats seulement désirent entreprendre une action à laquelle tous leurs partenaires européens ne souhaitent pas se joindre, ils peuvent conclure un «accord partiel» qui n'engage qu'eux-mêmes.

Accord partiel dans le domaine social et de la santé publique

C'est ainsi que fut conclu, en 1959, par le Comité des Ministres du Conseil de l'Europe, l'Accord partiel dans le domaine social et de la santé publique, accord révisé par le Comité des Ministres en 1996 avec effet à partir du 1er janvier 1997. Les Etats suivants sont Membres de l'Accord Partiel: Autriche, Belgique, Chypre, Danemark, Finlande, France, Allemagne, Irlande, Italie, Luxembourg, Pays-Bas, Norvège, Portugal, Slovénie, Espagne, Suède, Suisse et Royaume-Uni de Grande-Bretagne et d'Irlande du Nord.

Le but des activités de santé publique de l'Accord partiel est de protéger le consommateur des risques potentiels liés au mode de vie d'aujourd'hui. Les comités d'experts établissent les bases scientifiques de réglementations nationales et internationales concernant des produits qui ont un impact direct ou indirect sur la chaîne alimentaire humaine (contrôle de denrées alimentaires, nutrition, sécurité alimentaire, santé du consommateur, matériaux entrant en contact avec les denrées alimentaires, matières aromatisantes), les pesticides, les produits pharmaceutiques et les produits cosmétiques.

Le Comité directeur responsable des activités concernant la protection sanitaire du consommateur est le Comité de Santé publique, qui est composé de hauts fonctionnaires des ministères de la Santé des divers Etats membres. Il supervise les activités des Comités d'experts et dicte les principes généraux de la politique de santé publique que ces comités d'experts devront appliquer dans leurs travaux.

L'Accord partiel a toujours suivi de près l'évolution des techniques et des progrès scientifiques, et les résolutions, lignes directrices et rapports qui résultent de ses travaux sont souvent pionniers dans les domaines touchés.

Dans la plupart des domaines, l'approche est celle de l'évaluation des groupes de substances chimiques, l'établissement de spécifications techniques et technologiques, l'élaboration de taux maximaux et indiqués et la préparation de listes inventaires de substances chimiques.

Introduction

A few years ago the Committee of Experts on Cosmetic Products drew attention to 300 plants and their preparations used in cosmetic products.

The first volume of the publication contains 71 datasheets and this second volume presents a further 44.

The system used to classify the plants and plant preparations has been slightly modified, the three categories now being:

Category A: "Plants and plant preparations that can be used in cosmetic products". This category groups together ingredients which have been evaluated on the basis of available data. Based on those data, no health hazards have been demonstrated for the ingredients. In principle, and providing the stated applications and concentrations are respected, their use in cosmetic products is therefore considered as safe. Where appropriate, recommendations are made concerning specific constituents;

Category B: "Plants and plant preparations it has not been possible to evaluate". This category groups together plants and plant preparations in respect of which the Committee of Experts needs further information before it can give a confirmed opinion regarding their safety-in-use;

Category C: "Plants and plant preparations which it is recommended should not be used in cosmetic products". This category groups together plants and plant preparations which may pose a health risk and are therefore not recommended for use in cosmetic products.

Introduction

Il y a quelques années, le Comité d'experts sur les produits cosmétiques a appelé l'attention sur 300 plantes et leurs préparations susceptibles d'être utilisées dans les produits cosmétiques.

Le premier volume de cette publication contient 71 monographies. Ce deuxième volume présente 44 nouvelles monographies.

Le système de classification des plantes et préparations à base de plantes a été légèrement modifié. Désormais, les trois catégories sont:

- **catégorie A «plantes et préparations à base de plantes qui peuvent être utilisées dans les produits cosmétiques»:** cette catégorie rassemble les ingrédients qui ont pu être évalués à partir des données disponibles et ne présentent pas de danger pour la santé. Leur utilisation dans les produits cosmétiques est donc, en principe, sans risque pour les applications citées et aux concentrations indiquées. Le cas échéant, des recommandations sont formulées à propos des composants spécifiques;

- **catégorie B «plantes et préparations à base de plantes qui n'ont pu être évaluées»:** cette catégorie réunit les plantes et préparations à base de plantes pour lesquelles le comité d'experts a besoin d'informations supplémentaires avant de pouvoir formuler un avis confirmé sur leur sécurité d'utilisation;

- **catégorie C «plantes et préparations à base de plantes qu'il est recommandé de ne pas utiliser dans les produits cosmétiques»:** cette catégorie réunit les plantes et préparations de plantes susceptibles de présenter un danger pour la santé, et qu'il n'est donc pas recommandé d'utiliser dans les produits cosmétiques.

Datasheets

Acorus calamus

Botanical name[1]	*Acorus calamus* L. (var. *americanus* Rafin.)
Botanical synonyms[1,2]	*Acorus calamus* var. *angustifolius* Schott, *Acorus aromaticus* Gilib., *Acorus. belangeri* Schott, *Acorus casia* Bertol., *Acorus. griffithii* Schott, *Acorus odoratus* Lamk., *Acorus spurius* Schott, *Acorus terrestris* Spreng., *Oronthium cochinchinensis* Lour.
Botanical family	Araceae

Common names

Sweet flag	(English)
Kalmoes	(Dutch)
Kalmojuuri	(Finnish)
Acore	(French)
Kalmus	(German)
Calamo aromatico	(Italian)
Kalmusrot	(Norwegian)
Cálamo aromático	(Spanish)
Kalmus	(Swedish)

EU INCI name[3]	*Acorus calamus*
CTFA INCI name[4]	*Calamus (Acorus calamus)* extract

CAS number	84775-39-3
EINECS number	283-869-0
Parts used	Rhizomes

Important constituents including active principles[13,16,17]
- Essential oil (1.5-3.5%)[13]:
  Monoterpenes (methylisoeugenol (1%)[16], eugenol (0.3%)[16], methyleugenol, α- and β-pinene, camphene, α-phellandrene, myrcene, α-terpinene, limonene, β-ocymene, α-bergamoptene, camphor, cineole, linalool, bornyl acetate, terpinen-4-ol)
  Sesquiterpenes (β-,α- and γ-asarone[26], calamene (4%)[16], calamenol (5%)[16], calamone (1%)[16], b-pharnesene, δ-cadinene, β- and δ-elemene, β-selinene, shyobunone, α-copaene, α-cadinol, acorenone, acorone, isoacorone, acoragermacrone, acolamone, isoacolamone)
  Hydrocarbons (1,6-dimethyl-4-(1-methyl ethyl)-3,4,4a,7-tetrahydronaphthalene, calameone, preisocalamendiol, isocalamendiol)
  Aldehydes (acoradin and asarylaldehyde)
  Phenyl indane[24]
- Acorin, acoretin (choline)
- Tannins (1%)[17]

– Starch (25-40 %)[16.]

– Amino acids (arginine, lysine, phenylalanine,threonine,thrypto-phan)

– Triglycerides (cont. myristic, palmitic, palmitoleic, stearic, oleic, linoleic, arachic acids)

– Sugars (maltose, glucose, fructose)

– Resin (2.5)[16.]

– Gum

Note. The Acorus calamus americanus does not contain β-asarone[13., 16., 19.]

The Chinese and Indian varieties can contain up to 85 % of β-asarone in the essential oil[13.]

Preparation

1) Essential oil (var. americanus)
2) Calamus root extract[6.]

Manufacturing process

1) Steam distillation
2) Percolation with ethanol solution and concentration under vacuum

Examples of specifications

1)[11.] Specific gravity at 15°C: 0.950 to 0.974
Specific optical rotation: +13° 48′ to + 15°
Refraction index at 20°C: 0.5013 to 1.5069
Saponification index: 8.4 to 10.7
Solubility: soluble in 0.5-5 vol. alcohol 90%

2)[6.] pH (c=10, water): 3.7-4.7
Specific gravity at 20°C: 0.900-1.000
Heavy metal: not more than 10 ppm
Arsenic: not more than 2 ppm
Residue on evaporation: 0.4-1.0 w/v% (10 ml, 105° C, 6-hours)

Intended cosmetic effects and used concentration in cosmetic products

Tonic, refreshing, astringent, soothing; fragrance
Hair tonics, antidandruff products, mouthwashes and toothpastes, stimulant bath preparations and shampoos, emulsions for massage

Up to 0.4% in fragrances

Other possible effects[13.]

Anti-inflammatory, anti-oedema, granulation promoting agent, anti-microbial[16.], lipolytic (traditional)[13.], insect repellent (traditional)[13.]

Main toxicological data[23.]

LD_{50}, oral in rats: 777 mg/kg b.w.
888 mg/kg b.w.
LD_{50}, dermal in guinea pigs: > 5000 mg/kg b.w.
LD_{50}, i.p. in rats: 221 mg/kg b.w. (A stem volatile fraction of roots and rhizomes Indian variety oil tested)
LD_{50}, i.p. in mice: 400 mg were toxic (An oleoresin Indian variety oil tested)
Subchronic toxicity: oral in rats: 2 500, 5 000 and 10 000 ppm fed for 18 weeks, depressed growth and caused liver changes; severity

of effects decreased at lower dose levels. Heart changes with varying degrees of necrosis of muscle fibre, early fibrosis and infiltration with mononuclear cells, were also observed at all dose levels tested.

Acute eye irritation: no data

Primary skin irritation: non-irritant when tested at 4% in petrolatum after a 48-hour closed-patch test on human subjects and on mice, swine, rabbits and guinea pigs

Sensitisation animals: no data

Sensitisation man: Skin erythema and contact dermatitis in hypersensitive individuals using bath preparations containing calamus oil have been reported. No sensitisation reaction has been reported in 23 volunteers undergoing a maximisation test at 4% calamus oil in petrolatum nor in 250 patients with dermatitis or known to be reactive to other allergens

Undesirable active principles:

(β-asarone)

Carcinogenic in rodents, inducing tumours of the liver and small intestine.

Contradictory results on mutagenic activity *in vitro* with S 9 mix activation[27.]

(Methyleugenol)

Carcinogenic in preweaned mice, inducing liver tumours

Mutagenic in several systems[28.]

(Eucalyptol or 1,8-cineole or p-cineole)

has been studied sub-chronically in rats and mice; a NOEL of 300 mg/kg bw has been established. Eucalyptol has been found non mutagenic in different systems[29.]

Databases used	CA Search 1967-95, Medline 1966-95, Embase 1974-95, Ref. Tox. Eff. Chem. Sub.
Keywords	Acorus calamus
Evaluation and remarks	**Cat. C – (if detectable levels of β-asarone or methyleugenol are present)** **Cat. B – (if detectable levels of β-asarone and methyleugenol are not present)**

General references

1. Index Kewensis, Clarendon Press
2. Penso G., Index Plantarum Medicinalium Totius Mundi Eorumque Synonymorum, OEMF, 1983
3. European Commission Decision 96/335/EC of 8 May 1996, Official Journal of the European Community No. L132 of 1 June 1996
4. International Cosmetic Ingredient Dictionary 6th ed., CTFA, 1, 1995
5. Benigni R., Capra C., Cattorini P.E., Piante Medicinali chimica farmacologia e terapia, Inverni & Della Beffa, 1, 181-184, 1971
6. Comprehensive Licensing Standards of Cosmetics by Category, Yakuji Nippo Ltd., 6, 90, 1992

7. Council of Europe, Flavouring substances and natural sources of flavourings 3rd ed. Maisonneuve, (13 N3), 1981
8. Flavouring Extract Manufactures Association (Fema), Survey of flavouring ingredients usage levels, (No. 2226, 2227), Food Technology, 163 (265), 1965
9. Fenaroli G., Sostanze Aromatiche Naturali, Hoepli, 424, 1963
10. Grieve M., A modern herbal, Barnes & Noble Books, 726-729, 1996
11. Guenther E., The essential oils, D. Van Nostrand, 4, 109, 1952
12. The Japanese Cosmetic Ingredients Codex, Yakuji Nippo, Ltd, 119, 1993
13. Leung A.Y., Foster S, Encyclopedia of Common Natural Ingredients, Wiley & Son Publ., 111-113, 1996
14. Martindale 31st ed., The Royal Pharmaceutical Society, 1996
15. Merck Index 12th ed., Merck & Co. Inc., 1996
16. Newall C., Anderson L., Phillipson J.D., Herbal Medicines: a guide for health care professionals, The Pharmaceutical Press, 55-57, 1996
17. Proserpio G., Martelli A., Patri G.F., Elementi di fitocosmesi, Sepem, 2, 581-582, 1983
18. Van Hellemont J., Compendium de Phytotherapie, APB, 7-8, 1986
19. Wichtl M., Teedrogen, WVG, 260-262, 1989

Specific references

20. Arora R.C., Agarwal N., Arora S., Garg R.K., Acorus calamus – A lipid lowering agent, Zywienie Czlowieka I Metabolizm, 14, 2, 81-83, 1987
21. Chowdhury A.K.A., Ara T. et al., A new phenyl propane derivative from Acorus calamus, Pharmazie, 48, 786-787, 1993
22. Nater J.P., De Groot A.C., Unwanted effects of cosmetics and drugs used in dermatology, Excerpta Medica, 316-317, 1983
23. Opdyke. D.L.J., Food and Cosmetics Toxicology, 15, 623, 1977
24. Saxena D.B., Phenyl Indane from Acorus calamus, Phytochem. 25, 2, 553-555, 1986
25. Shimizu M., Matsuzawa T., Hase K. et al., Studies on Bathing Agent I. Anti-inflammatory Effect of Bathing Agent Used for Skin Disease, Shoyakugaku Zasshi, 47, 1, 1-4, 1993
26. IFRA - International Fragrance Association, Code of Practice, cis and trans-Asarone monograph, Dec. 1991
27. Recommendations concerning undesirable active principles, 3.2, 28th meeting, Rome, Committee of Experts on Cosmetic Products, 3-7 November 1997, Council of Europe
28. Recommendations concerning undesirable active principles, 3.11, 28th meeting, Rome, Committee of Experts on Cosmetic Products, 3-7 November 1997, Council of Europe
29. Recommendations concerning undesirable active principles, 3.8, 28th meeting, Rome, Committee of Experts on Cosmetic Products, 3-7 November 1997, Council of Europe
30. DAB 6
31. Ph B II
32. Ph Ned F 6
33. Ph. Helv. VII
34. OAB IX

Artemisia absinthium

Botanical name[1]	*Artemisia absinthium* Tourn. ex L.
Botanical synonyms[2]	*Absinthium officinale* Brot., *Artemisia vulgare* Lam.
Botanical family	Asteraceae
Common names	Wormwood, Mugwort (English)
	Alsem (Dutch)
	Mali (Finnish)
	Absinthe grande (French)
	Wermut, Wermutkraut (German)
	Assenzio (Italian)
	Malurt (Norwegian)
	Absenta (Spanish)
	Malört (Swedish)
EU INCI name[3]	*Artemisia absinthium*
CTFA INCI name[4]	Mugwort (*Artemisia absinthium*) extract

CAS number	84929-19-1 (*Artemisia absinthium*)
	84775-45-1 (*Artemisia vulgare*)
	546-80-5 (α-thujone)
	471-15-8 (β-thujone)
EINECS number	284-503-2 (*Artemisia absinthium*)
	283-874-8 (*Artemisia vulgare*)
Parts used	Leaves and flowering tops

Important constituents including active principles[11, 15, 16, 19]

- Essential oil (up to 1.7%)[11, 23]:
  Monoterpenes (α- and β-thujone, pinene, sabinene, phellandrene, camphene, myrcene, β-ocimene, thujylalcohol, thujyl acetate, cineole, sabinol, terpinen-4-ol, linalol, geraniol, nerol)
  Sesquiterpenes (β-caryophyllene, cadinene, bisabolene)
  Azulenes (chamazulene up to 17%[11], 3,6-dihydrochamazulene, 5,6- diydrochamazulene)
  Diterpenes[25]
  Sesquiterpene lactones[26, 27] (absinthin, anabsinthin, artabsin, artemetin, arabsin, artabin, ketopelenolide A, artanolide, artemoline, artenolide, anabsin, matricine, isoabsinthin and absintholide)
  Polyol (quebrachitol)
- Flavonoids[22] (quercetin-3-glucoside, rutin, isorhamnetin-3-glucoside, isorhamnetin-3-rhamnoglucoside, patuletin-3-glucoside,

patuletin-3-rhamnoglucoside, spinacetin-3-glucoside, spinacetin-3-rhamnoglucoside)
– Coumarins
– Phenol acids
– Phytosterols[20.]
– Oligosaccharides[28.] (inulobiose)
– Carotene (0.05%)[11.]
– Vitamin C (up to 0.26%)[11.]
– Tannins (up to 7.7%)[11.]

Preparation
1) Essential oil
2) Hydroalcoholic fluid extract

Manufacturing process
1) Steam distillation
2) Extraction with alcohol 20% and concentration under vacuum to final E/D ratio 1:1

Examples of specifications
1)[8.] Specific gravity at 20°: 0.918-0.943
Acid Number: up to 5.6
Ester Number: 15-37
Solubility: in 1 to 2-vol. of alcohol 80%

Intended cosmetic effects and used concentration in cosmetic products
Tonic, stimulant, fragrance
(Essential oil)
Up to 0.01% in detergents.
Up to 0.03% in creams, lotions

Other possible effects
Anti-microbial, vulnerary[15.], rubifacient, anti-inflammatory

Main toxicological data
(Thujone) is toxic
(Essential oil)[21., 24.]
LD_{50} oral in rats: 960 mg/kg
LD_{50} dermal in rabbits: > 5000 mg/kg
Skin irritation in hairless mice: (undiluted) not irritating in rabbits: applied full strength to intact or abraded skin for 24-hour under occlusion, it was slightly irritating in humans: tested at 2% in petrolatum, it produced no irritation after a 48-hour closed-patch test
Sensitisation: A maximisation test was carried out on 25 volunteers. The material was tested at a concentration of 2% in petrolatum and produced no sensitisation reactions
Phototoxicity on hairless mice and swine: no phototoxic effects were reported for undiluted artemisia oil

(Extract)
LD_{50} i.p. in rats: 1000 mg/kg
Urine volume increased

(Eucalyptol or 1,8-cineole or p-cineole)
has been studied sub-chronically in rats and mice; a NOEL of 300 mg/kg bw has been established. Eucalyptol has been found non mutagenic in different systems[29.]

Databases used   CA Search 1967-95, Medline 1966-95, Embase 1974-95, Ref. Tox. Eff. Chem. Sub., Biosis, Toxline, Kosmet, Napralert, Cosmet

Keywords   *Artemisia absinthium,* Mugwort

Evaluation and remarks   Cat. C (essential oil)
Cat. A (Hydroalcoholic fluid extract)

The essential oil is neurotoxic owing to its lipophilethujone content. Transdermal penetration cannot be excluded. However, the thujone concentration in the fluid extract is weak and *a priori* should not cause any side effects

General references
1. Index Kewensis, Clarendon Press
2. Penso G., Index Plantarum Medicinalium Totius Mundi Eorumque Synonymorum, OEMF, 1983
3. European Commission Decision 96/335/EC of 8 May 1996, Official Journal of the European Community No. L132 of 1 June 1996
4. International Cosmetic Ingredient Dictionary 6th ed., CTFA, 1995
5. Benigni R., Capra C., Cattorini P.E., Piante Medicinali chimica farmacologia e terapia, Inverni & Della Beffa, 1, 118-121, 1971
6. Council of Europe, Flavouring substances and natural sources of flavourings 3rd ed. Maisonneuve, (61 N2), 1981
7. Flavouring Extract Manufacturers Association (Fema), Survey of flavouring ingredients usage levels, (Nos. 3114, 3115, 3116), Food Technology, 197 (299), 1965
8. Fenaroli G., Sostanze Aromatiche Naturali, Hoepli, 378-381, 1963
9. Grieve M., A modern herbal, Barnes & Noble Books, 858-860, 1996
10. Guenther E., The essential oils, D. Van Nostrand, 5, 487-496, 1952
11. Leung A.Y., Foster S, Encyclopedia of Common Natural Ingredients, Wiley & Son Publ., 1-4, 1996
12. Martindale 31st ed., The Royal Pharmaceutical Society, 1996
13. Merck Index 12th ed., Merck & Co. Inc., 1996
14. Monographs, Bundesanzeiger Absinthii herba, No. 228 (Dec. 5, 1984) and No. 122 (July 6, 1988), through Le monografie tedesche, Studio Edizioni, 1, 1994
15. Paris R.R., Moyse H., Matière Médicale, Masson, 3, 418-419, 1971
16; Van Hellemont J., Compendium de Phytotherapie, APB, 49-50, 1986
17. Wichtl M., Teedrogen, WVG, 528-531, 1989

Specific references
18. Beckstrom-Sternberg SM, Duke J.A., "The Phytochemical Database"
19. CE Datasheet Nov. 1996

20. Darwish Sayed M., Soliman F.M., El-Shamy, El-Shabrawy A.O., Sterols of *Artemisia absinthium* L., Egypt. J. Pharm. Sci., 19, 1-4, 232-327, 1978
21. Datasheet, RD 5/7-27, May 1997
22. Hoffmann B., Herrmann K., Flavonolglykoside des Beifuß (*Artemisia vulgaris* L.), Estragon (*Artemisia dracunculus* L.) und Wermut (*Artemisia absinthium* L.), Z. Lebensm Unters Forsch., 174, 211-215, 1982
23. Nin S., Arfaioli P., Bosetto M., Quantitative Determination of Some Essential Oil Components of Selected *Artemisia absinthium* Plants, J. Essent. Oil Res., 7, 271-277, 1995
24. Opdyke D.L.J., Food and Cosmetics Toxicology, 13S, 721, 1975
25. Rücker G., Manns D., Wilbert S., Homoditerpene Peroxides from *Artemisia absinthium,* Phytochemistry, 31, 1, 340-342, 1992
26. Von Schneider G. and Mielke B., Zur Analytik der Bitterstoffe Absinthin, Artabsin und Matrizin aus *Artemisia absinthium* L., Deutsche Apotheker Zeitung, 118, 13, 469-472, 1978
27. Von Schneider G. and Mielke B., Zur Analytik der Bitterstoffe Absinthin, Artabsin und Matrizin aus *Artemisia absinthium* L., Teil II: Isolierung und Gehaltsbestimmungen, Deutsche Apotheker Zeitung, 119, 13, 977-982, 1978
28. Tourn M.L. e Lombard A., Studi sugli oligofruttosani delle foglie di Artemisia Absinthium, Atti Cl. di Scienze fisiche, 108, 60, 941-950, 1974
29. Recommendations concerning undesirable active principles, 3.8, 28th meeting Committee of Experts on Cosmetic Products, Rome, 3-7 November 1997, Council of Europe.
30. DAB 10
31. OAB '83
32. Ph. Helv. VII
33. FU IX

Camellia japonica

Botanical name[1]	*Camellia japonica* L.
Botanical synonyms[2]	*Camelia japonica* L.
Botanical family	Theaceae
Common names	Camellia (English)
	Kamelia (Finnish)
	Kamelie (German)
	Camelia (Italian)
	Camelia (Spanish)
	Kamelia (Swedish)
EU INCI name	-
CTFA INCI name[3]	*Camellia japonica* extract

CAS number

EINECS number

Parts used   Seeds (sometimes leaves and fruits)

Important constituents including active principles
- Tannins (camelliatannins A,B,C, D, E, F, G)[5, 6, 7, 8]
- Triterpene saponins (camelliasaponins A1, A2, B1, B2, C1 and C2, camellidin I and II)[10, 13]
- Triglycerides (37-38%)[9]. (containing palmitic 8.3%, palmitoleic 0.1%, stearic 0.5%, oleic 86%, linoleic 3.1%, linolenic 0.1%, arachidic acids 0.9%)[11]
- Phytosterols (1% in the oil)[11]

Preparation
1) Camellia oil from seeds[12]
2) Camellia extract from seeds[14]

Manufacturing process
1) Extraction with hexane
2) Extraction with water of defatted seeds

Examples of specifications
1)[11] Specific gravity at 20°C: 0.9146
Refractive index at 20°C: 1,4682
Acid number: < 2
Iodine number: $\cong$ 80
Unsaponifiable: 1%
2)[4] Residue on ignition: not more than 3.0%
Heavy metals: not more than 20 ppm
Arsenic: not more than 2pp

Intended cosmetic effects and use concentration in cosmetic products
Emollient, conditioning in skin and hair cosmetics

Other possible effects Anti-inflammatory, anti-fungal

Main toxicological data Oil not used as food because it contain saponins[9].

Databases used CA Search 1967-97, Medline 1966-97, Embase 1974-97, Ref. Tox. Eff. Chem. Sub., Biosis, Toxline, Kosmet

Keywords *Camellia japonica,* Common *Camellia*

Evaluation and remarks **Cat. B (oil; extract)**

Despite the lack of toxicological data, it is reasonable to think that the seed oil contains only lipids and saponins; unfortunately there is no evidence that these are harmless.

General references

1. Index Kewensis, Clarendon Press
2. Penso G., Index Plantarum Medicinalium Totius Mundi Eorumque Synonymorum, OEMF, 1983
3. International Cosmetic Ingredient Dictionary 6th ed., CTFA, 1995
4. The Japanese Cosmetic Ingredients Codex, ed. Yakuji Nippo Ltd., 126, 1993

Specific references

5. Han L. Et al., Tannins of theaceous Plants. V. Camellitannins F, G and H, three New Tannins from Camellia japonica L., Chem. Pharm. Bull., *42*, 7, 1399-1409, 1994
6. Hatano T. et al., Tannins of theaceous Plants. III. Camellitannins A and B, Two New Complex Tanins from *Camellia japonica* L., Chem. Pharm. Bull., 39, 4, 876-880, 1991
7. Hatano T. et al., Camelliatannin D, A New Inhibitor of Bone Resorption, from *Camellia japonica*, Chem. Pharm. Bull., 43, 11, 2033-2035, 1995
8. Hatano T. et al., Tannins and Related Polyphenols of theaceous Plants. VIII. Camelliatannin D and E, New Complex Tannins from *Camellia japonica* Leaves, Chem. Pharm. Bull., 43, 10, 1629-1633, 1995
9. Martinenghi G.B., Tecnologia Chimica Industriale degli Oli, Grassi e Derivati, Hoepli, 429, 1963
10. Nagata T. et al., Camellidins, Anti-fungal Saponins Isolated from *Camellia japonica,* Agric. Biol. Chem., 49, 4, 1181-1186, 1985
11. Sabetay S., Bevon M.T., Produits de beauté cosmétiques et dermo-pharmaceutiques contenant de l'huile de camélia (Camélia japonica), Fr. Demande 2.051.902, 14 May 1971
12. Sabetay S., Bevon M.T., Produits de beauté cosmétiques et dermo-pharmaceutiques contenant de l'huile de camélia (Camélia japonica), Fr. Demande 2.196.147, 15 Mar 1974
13. Yoshikawa M. et al., Bioactive Saponins and Glycosides. V. Acylated Polyhydroxyolean-12-ene Triterpene Oligoglycosides, Camelliasaponins A_1, A_2, B_1, B_2, C_1 and C_2, Chem. Pharm. Bull., 44, 10, 1899-1907, 1996

Camellia sinensis

Botanical name[1]	*Camellia sinensis* Kuntze
Botanical synonyms[2]	*Camelia sinensis* Kuntze, *Camelia thea* Link., *Camelia theifera* Griff., *Thea bohea* L., *Thea cantoniensis* Lour., *Thea chinensis* Sims., *Thea chinensis* Sims. var. cantoniensis Pierre, *thea cochinchinensis* Lour., *Thea sinensis* L., *Thea viridis* L., *Theaphylla annamiensis* Raf., *Theaphylla cantoniensis* Raf.
Botanical family	Theaceae
Common names	Tea (English)
	Theestruik (Dutch)
	Vihreatee (Finnish)
	Théier (French)
	Teestrauch (German)
	Tè (Italian)
	Té (Spanish)
	Tebuske (Swedish)
EU INCI name[3]	*Camellia sinensis*
CTFA INCI name[4]	*Camellia sinensis* extract
	Camellia sinensis oil

CAS number	84650-60-2
	68916-73-4 (oil)
EINECS number	283-519-7
Parts used	Leaves, seeds

Important constituents including active principles[7, 9]

- Flavouring substances (over 300 compounds)[9]
- Xantines (caffeine (1-5%)[9], theobromine, theophylline, adenine, xanthine, dimethylxanthine)
- Polyphenols (5-27%)[9]
  Flavanols (cathechin, epicathechin, gallocathechin, epigallo-cathechin, epicathechingallate, epigallocathechingallate)
  Procyanidins
  Phenol acids (gallic and chlorogenic acids)
  Flavonoids (quercetin, quercitrin, rutin, kaempferol, myricetin, apigenin, luteolin)
  Tannins
- Triterpene saponins
- Mineral salts (4-7%)[19] (F, Al, K, Mn)

– Fatty acids (4-16.5%)[9] (oleic 83.3-86.7%, linoleic 6.8-10%, palmitic 4.9-7.6%, stearic 0.8-1.2%, arachidic 0.6-0.8%)[16, 18, 19]
– Organic acids (malic, succinic, oxalic acids)
– Phytosterols (a-spinasterol, stigmasterol)
– Vitamins (C, B_1, B_2, B_3)
– Amino acids
– Proteins (12-15%)[9] (mainly albumines)
– Sugars (1-2%)[9]
– Polysaccharides
– Pectines

Preparation
1) Dry extract[20]
2) Tea extract[5]
3) Oil[11]

Manufacturing process
1) Percolation with water and concentration by spray drying to dryness.
2) Dry-distill the branches and leaves under reduced pressure. To 1 part of the fraction add 4 parts of glycerine and 20 parts of purified water.
3) Extraction of leaves with hexane

Examples of specifications
1)[20] pH (1% in water): 4.5-6.5
    Sulfated ash: ≤10.0% Water (acc. K.Fischer): ≤6.0%
2)[5] pH: 4.0-6.0
    Specific gravity at 20°C: 0.959-1.000
    Heavy metals: not more than 20 ppm
    Arsenic: nor more than 2 ppm
    Residue on evaporation: 0.5-3.0%
3)[11] Acid value: < not more than 0.5
    Iodine value: 80-90
    Saponification value: 185-195
    Unsaponifiable matter: not more than 1.5%
    Purity: Dissolve 1.0 g of tea seed oil in 10 ml of ether: the solution is clear.

Intended cosmetic effects and use concentration in cosmetic products

Tonic, astringent, flavouring, protectant.
Emollient, moisturising, conditioner.
Concentration limited for dry and damaged hair and scalp shampoos and conditioning products, nail strengtheners, after-sun products, eye contour products, hand creams, moisturising products for dry, ageing skin.

Other possible effects
Hemostatic[9], stimulant, antibacterial (oil)

Main toxicological data
(Extract) [RTECS]
LD_{50} oral in mice: 3900 mg/kg
LD_{50} i.p. in mice: 316 mg/kg
Hypoglycemia. Effect on inflammation or mediation of inflammation

(Oil)

Acute toxicity: no toxic effects are known[19.]

(Tannins) [(RTECS)]

Neoplastic by RTECS criteria. Tumours at site of application TDL_0 subcutaneous in rat: 1850 mg/kg

Databases used

CA Search 1967-97, Medline 1966-97, Embase 1974-97, Ref. Tox. Eff. Chem. Sub., Biosis, Toxline, Kosmet

Keywords

Camellia sinensis, Thea, Thea sinensis, Tea

Evaluation and remarks

Cat. A (dry extract; tea extract)
Cat. B (oil)

Although there are no toxicological data for external use, it seems reasonable to think that the extracts, which are likely to be rich in polyphenols, are atoxic. On the other hand, the oil may contain saponins, the possible side-effects of which are not known.

General references

1. Index Kewensis, Clarendon Press
2. Penso G., Index Plantarum Medicinalium Totius Mundi Eorumque Synonymorum, OEMF, 1983
3. European Commission Decision 96/335/EC of 8 May 1996, Official Journal of the European Community No. L132 of 1 June 1996
4. International Cosmetic Ingredient Dictionary 6th ed., CTFA, 1995
5. Comprehensive Licensing Standards of Cosmetics by Category, Yakuji Nippo Ltd., 5, 270-271,1990
6. Council of Europe, Flavouring substances and natural sources of flavourings 3rd ed. Maisonneuve, (451, N 2), 1981
7. Fenaroli G., Sostanze Aromatiche Naturali, Hoepli, 933-934, 1963
8. Grieve M., A modern herbal, Barnes & Noble Books, 792-793, 1996
9. Leung A.Y., Foster S, Encyclopedia of Common Natural Ingredients, Wiley & Son Publ., 489-492, 1996
10. Martindale 31st ed., The Royal Pharmaceutical Society, 1996
11. The Japanese Cosmetic Ingredients Codex, ed. Yakuji Nippo Ltd., 870, 1993
12. Paris R.R., Moyse H., Matière Mèdicale, Masson 2nd ed., 237-245, 1981
13. Proserpio G., Martelli A., Patri G.F., Elementi di fitocosmesi, Sepem, 2, 560-561, 1983
14. Van Hellemont J., Compendium de Phytotherapie, APB, 394-395, 1986
15. Wichtl M., Teedrogen, WVG, 492-494, 1989

Specific references

16. Bhuyan L.P. and Mahanta P.K., Studies on fatty acids composition in Tea Camellia sinensis, J. Sci Food Agric 46, 325-330, 1989

17. Liang Y.R., Liu Z.S., Xu Y.R., Hu Y.L., A study on chemical composition of two special green teas (*Camellia sinensis*), J. Sci Food Agric 53, 541-548, 1990
18. Owuor P.O., Plucking standard effects and the distribution of fatty acids in the tea (*Camellia sinensis* L.) Leaves, Food Chemistry, 37, 27-35, 1990
19. Technical documentation Alban Muller international, Camellia oil
20. Indena Product Specification

Centaurea cyanus

Botanical name[1]	*Centaurea cyanus* L.
Botanical synonyms	-
Botanical family	Asteraceae
Common names	Cornflower (English)
	Korenbloem (Dutch)
	Bleuet des champs (French)
	Kornblume (German)
	Fiordaliso (Italian)
	Kornblomst (Norwegian)
	Azulejo (Spanish)
EU INCI name[2]	*Centaurea cyanus*
CTFA INCI name[3]	Cornflower (*Centaurea cyanus*)
	Cornflower (*Centaurea cyanus*) extract

CAS number	84012-18-0
	68916-70-1
EINECS number	281-664-0
Parts used	Flowers

Important constituents including active principles[11]

- Phenol acids[14] (chlorogenic, cis- and trans-caffeic, p-hydroxybenzoic, p-coumaric, vanillic, syringic, ferulic, salicylic, p-hydroxyphenylacetic, o-hydroxyphenylacetic, cis and trans-sinapic and benzoic acids)
- Flavonoids (quercimetrin, apiin, apigenin 4'-O-β-D-glucoside 7-O- β-D-glucuronide, centaurein)
- Coumarins (scopoletin, umbelliferone)
- Anthocyanidins (cyanidin 3-succinyl glucoside 5-glucoside, cicorine, pelarqinine 3.5%[11])
- Anthoxanthins
- Catechins (gallocatechin)
- Tannins
- Amino acids – Thiophene derivatives[15].
- Sugars (glucose, fructose, saccharose and raffinose), mucilages, pectins
- Mineral salts
- Sesquiterpene lactones (swertiamarin)
- C_{13}-C_{17} polyunsaturated hydrocarbons and alcohols

Preparation[12]

1) Hydroglycolic extract
2) Distilled water

Manufacturing process[12]

1) Percolation with propylene glycol 50% to final E/D ratio 10:1
2) Distillation in steam current to final W/D ratio 2:1

Examples of specifications[12]

1) pH: 5.2 - 6.1
   Specific gravity at 20°C: 1.039 - 1.043
   Refractive index at 20°C: 1.338 - 1.394
   Dry residue: 0.40 - 1.00
   Heavy metals: not more than 5 ppm
2) Density at 20°C: 1.035 - 1.040
   Refractive index at 20°C: 1.386 at 1.390

Intended cosmetic effects and used concentration in cosmetic products

Tonic, soothing, astringent and refreshing (tannins), moisturising (mucilages)

(hydroglycolic extract)
Up to 5%

(distilled water)
Up to 50% in cleansing lotions, gels and other cosmetic products for eye contour, masks, detergents and pre- and after-shave products for sensitive skin

Other possible effects

Mild anti-inflammatory, antiseptic in eye drops, free radical scavenger.

Main toxicological data[12]

Mixture of distilled waters containing 5%:[16]
Primary skin irritation on rabbits: non-irritant
Acute eye irritation on rabbits: non-irritant

Databases used

CA Search 1967-95, Medline 1966-95, Embase 1974-95, Ref. Tox. Eff. Chem. Sub.

Keywords

Centaurea cyanus

Evaluation and remarks

Cat. B

General references

1. Index Kewensis, Clarendon Press
2. European Commission Decision 96/335/EC of 8 May 1996, Official Journal of the European Community No. L132 of 1 June 1996
3. International Cosmetic Ingredient Dictionary 6th ed., CTFA, 1, 1995
4. Cosmetic Licensing Standards of Cosmetics by Category, Yakuji Nippo Ltd., 2, 163, 1987
5. Council of Europe, Flavouring substances and natural sources of flavourings 3rd ed. Maisonneuve, (119,N2), 1981
6. Grieve M., A modern herbal, Barnes & Noble Books, 223-224, 1996
7. The Japanese Cosmetic Ingredients Codex, ed. Yakuji Nippo Ltd., 175-176, 1993

8. Monographs Cyani flos, Bundesanzeiger, No. 43 (Mar. 02,1989) through Le monografie tedesche, Studio Edizioni, 4,1996
9. Paris R.R., Moyse H., Matière Médicale, Masson ed., 3, 454, 1971
10. Proserpio G., Martelli A., Patri G.F., Elementi di fitocosmesi, Sepem, 2, 1983
11. Van Hellemont J., Compendium de Phytotherapie, APB, 90,1986

Specific references

12. Indena Product Specification
13. Nater J.P., De Groot A.C., Unwanted effects of cosmetic and drugs used in dermatology, Excerpta Medica, 314- 318, 1983
14. Swiatek L., Zadernowski R., Occurence of aromatic acids and sugars in flowers of Centaurea cyanus L., through Chem. Abstr. 120, 158782n, 1994
15. Tosi B., Bonora A., Dall'Olio G., Bruni A., Screening for toxic-thiophene compounds from crude drugs of the family compositae used in northern Italy, Phyto therapy research, 5, 2, 59-62, 1991
16. Indena's reports

Chondrus crispus

Botanical name	*Chondrus crispus* (L.) Stack.
Botanical synonyms[1]	*Fucus crispus* L.
Botanical family	Gigartinaceae
Common names	Carrageen, Irish moss (English)
	Iers mos (Dutch)
	Irlannin Levä (Finnish)
	Carragheen (French)
	Irländisches Moos (German)
	Carragenina (Italian)
	Carragaen (Spanish)
	Karragentang (Swedish)
EU INCI name[2]	*Chondrus crispus*
CTFA INCI name[3]	Carrageenan (*Chondrus crispus*)
	Carrageenan (*Chondrus crispus*) extract

CAS number	78005-48-8
	9000-07-1 (carrageenan)
EINECS number	305-775-1 (*Fucus crispus*)
	232-524-2 (carrageenan)
Parts used	Dried thalli

Important constituents including active principles[8]

- Sulfated polysaccharides 50-80%[12], containing galactanes up to 44% and sulfates up to 35% (Carrageenan: κ-form 25-30% degree of sulphation, λ-form 32-39% degree of sulphation, ι-form 28-35% degree of sulphation)[10, 12]
- Phospholipids
- Glycolipids
- Glycosylglycerides (mono-, di-galactosyl- and sulphoquinosyl- diacylglycerols)[14]
- Fatty acids (mainly palmitic, oleic, arachidonic, eicosapentanoic acids)
- Mineral salts (iodine, bromine, phosphorus, nitrogen)[13]

Preparation	Carrageenan
Manufacturing process	Extraction of dried thallus with hot alkaline water and precipitation with alcohol

Examples of specifications[7.]   pH (1% solution): 6.5-9.5
Lead: the limit is not more than 8 ppm
Arsenic: the limit is not more than 2 ppm
Loss on drying: not more than 10.0%

Intended cosmetic effects and use concentration in cosmetic products
Moisturising. Soothing.
Rheological additive, emulsifier
In toothpastes, hand lotions, creams for sensitive skin

Other possible effects   Thickening, emulsifying agent, bulk-forming agent, demulcent

Main toxicological data   ((δ–Carrageenan)[10.]
LD_{50} oral, in rats: > 5000 mg/kg
LD_{50} dermal, in rabbits: > 2000 mg/kg
LC_{50} (4 hr) in rats: > 930.8 ± 74.4 mg/m^3

(Carrageenan) [(RTECS)]
TDL_0 oral, in rats: 2.1 mg/kg/40 W
TDL_0 subcutaneous, in rats: 525 mg/kg/21 W
TDL_0 paren., in rats: 430 mg/kg
TD paren., in rats: 320 mg/kg
LDL_0 i.v., in rabbits: 5 mg/kg
LDL_0 i.v., in guinea pigs: 20 mg/kg
Carcinogenicity: no data are available for humans. Inadequate evidence of carcinogenicity in animals. Overall evaluation: group 3:this agent is not classifiable as to its carcinogenicity in humans [(HSDB)]

Databases used   CA Search 1967-97, Medline 1966-97, Embase 1974-97, Ref. Tox. Eff. Chem. Sub., Biosis, Toxline, Kosmet, HSDB

Keywords   *Chondrus crispus* or *fucus crispus*

Evaluation and remarks   **Cat. A (Carrageenans)**

Carrageenan has the capacity to form gels, the properties of which depend on the polysaccharide structure. These molecules have no toxic effects.

General references   1. Penso G., Index Plantarum Medicinalium Totius Mundi Eorumque Synonymorum, OEMF, 1983
2. European Commission Decision 96/335/EC of 8 May 1996, Official Journal of the European Community No. L132 of 1 June 1996
3. International Cosmetic Ingredient Dictionary 6th ed., CTFA, 1995
4.Council of Europe, Flavouring substances and natural sources of flavourings 3rd ed. Maisonneuve, (125 N2), 1981
5. Flavouring Extract Manufactures Association (Fema), Survey of flavouring ingredients usage levels, (No. 2596), Food Technology, 177 (279), 1965
6. Grieve M., A modern herbal, Barnes & Noble Books, 552, 1996
7. The Japanese Standards of Cosmetic Ingredients, second edition, Yakuji Nippo, Ltd, 73-74, 1985.

8. Leung A.Y., Foster S, Encyclopedia of Common Natural Ingredients, Wiley & Son Publ., 124-127, 1996
9. Martindale 31st ed., The Royal Pharmaceutical Society, 1996
10. Merck Index 12th ed., Merck & Co. Inc., 1996
11. Proserpio G., Martelli A., Patri G.F., Elementi di fitocosmesi, Sepem, 2, 808, 1983
12. Van Hellemont J., Compendium de Phytotherapie, APB, 167-168, 1986

Specific references

13. Chopin T., Lehmal H., Halcrow K., Polyphospates in the red macroalga *Chondrus crispus* (Rhodophyceae), New Phytol., *135*, 587-594, 1997
14. Pettitt T.R., Jones A.L., Harwood J.L., Lipids of the marine red algae, *Chondrus crispus* and *Polysiphonia lanosa*, Phytochemistry, 28, 2, 399-405, 1989

Citrus limon (L.) Burm (fruits)

Botanical name[1]	*Citrus limon* (L.) Burm.
Botanical synonyms[2]	*Citrus medica* L., *Citrus limonum* (Risso) Wight et Arn.
Botanical family	Rutaceae
Common names	Lemon (English)
	Zitroen (Dutch)
	Citron (French)
	Zitrone (German)
	Limone (Italian)
	Sitron (Norwegian)
	Limón (Spanish)
	Citron (Swedish)
EU INCI name[3]	*Citrus limonum*
CTFA INCI name[4]	Lemon (*Citrus medica limonum*) extract
	Lemon (*Citrus medica limonum*) juice
	Lemon (*Citrus medica limonum*) juice extract
	Lemon (*Citrus medica limonum*) juice powder
	Lemon (*Citrus medica limonum*) peel extract

CAS number	84929-31-7 (extract)
	68916-88-1 (juice)
EINECS number	284-515-8
Parts used	Fruits

Important constituents including active principles[12, 16, 17]

- Essential oil: (see monograph)
- Flavonoids (hesperidin, neohesperidin, naringin, diosmin, eriodictrin, eriocitrin, poncirin, limocitrol, limocitrin, quercetin[27], rutin)
- Coumarins (5-geranoxypsoralen, 8-geranoxypsoralen, byakangelicine, 5,7-dimethoxycoumarine)
- α-Hydroxyacids (citric, tartaric and malic acids) (6-10%)[16]
- Vitamins A, B, C (0.05%)[16]
- Bitter principle (Limonin)
- Phytosterols (β- and γ-sitosterol)
- Phenylpropanoid glycosides
- Pectin (10%)[16]
- Sugars (1.5%)[16] (fructose, glucose, sucrose)
- Stachydrine
- Amino acids
- Inositol

Preparation	1)[6] Lemon extract 2)[7] Lemon juice powder 3) Pectin
Manufacturing process	1)[6] Extraction of the fruits with purified water, glycerin, 1,3 buty-lene glycol, propylene glycol or a mixture of these; concentration of the extract and addition of concentrated glycerin 2)[7] By drying the fruit juice prepared by compressing or compressing and filtering 3) Extraction with water at pH 1.5-3.0 and 60-100°C followed with concentration and spray drying
Examples of specifications	1)[6] Heavy metals: not more than 20 ppm Arsenic: not more than 2 ppm 2)[7] Heavy metals: not more than 20 ppm Arsenic: not more than 2 ppm 3)[11] pH: 3.5-5.0 Heavy metals: not more than 22 ppm Arsenic: not more than 2 ppm Loss on drying: not more than 2.0% Residue on ignition: not more than 0.2%

Intended cosmetic effects and used concentration in cosmetic products

(Extract)
Tonic, refreshing, astringent, lightening, purifying, anti-ageing; flavour
Up to 5% in solutions, emulsions and gels for oily and impure skin, ageing skin
Pre- and after-sun products, mouthwashes and gargles for sensitive gums and oral mucosae

(Pectin)
Thickening agent

Other possible effects	Antimicrobial (pectin), anti-itching, free radical scavenger, anti-oedema, microvessel protectant
Main toxicological data	GRAS Status
Databases used	CA Search 1967-95, Medline 1966-96, Embase 1974-95, Ref. Tox. Eff. Chem. Sub., Toxline, IPA, Napralert, Cosmet Database
Keywords	*Citrus limon*
Evaluation and remarks	**Cat. A (extract; powder; pectin)** **Lemon juice powder and extract contain no more than traces of essential oil, including limonene and citral. *A priori*, therefore, sensitisation and allergy effects are not to be feared. Pectin is totally safe to use.**
General references	1. Index Kewensis, Clarendon Press 2. Penso G., Index Plantarum Medicinalium Totius Mundi Eorumque Synonymorum, OEMF, 1983

3. European Commission Decision 96/335/EC of 8 May 1996, Official Journal of the European Community No. L132 of 1 June 1996
4. International Cosmetic Ingredient Dictionary 6th ed. CTFA, 1, 1995
5. Benigni R., Capra C., Cattorini P.E., Piante Medicinali chimica farmacologia e terapia, Inverni & Della Beffa, 2, 1, 828-839, 1964
6. Comprehensive Licensing Standards of Cosmetics by Category, Yakuji Nippo Ltd., 1, 152, 1986
7. Comprehensive Licensing Standards of Cosmetics by Category, Yakuji Nippo Ltd., 5, 236, 1990
8. Council of Europe, Flavouring Substances and natural sources of flavourings 3rd ed. Maisonneuve, (139, N1),1981
9. Flavouring Extract Manufactures Association (Fema), Survey of flavouring ingredients usage levels, (No. 2623), Food Technology, 178 (280), 1965
10. Grieve M., A modern herbal, Barnes & Noble Books, 2, 474-476, 1996
11. Japanese Cosmetic Ingredients Codex, Yakuji Nippo, LTD., 440-441, 552, 1993
12. Leung A.Y., Foster S., Encyclopedia of common natural ingredients, Wiley & Son Publ., 342-344,1995
13. Martindale 31st ed., The Royal Pharmaceutical Society, 1996
14. Merck Index 12th ed., Merck & Co. Inc., 1996
15. Paris R.R., Moyse H., Matière Médicale 2nd ed., Masson, 2, 300, 1981
16. Proserpio G., Martelli A., Patri G.F., Elementi di fitocosmesi, Sepem, 2, 454-455, 1983
17. Van Hellemont J., Compendium de Phytotherapie, APB, 104-106, 1986
18. Wichtl M., Teedrogen, WVG, 538-539, 1989

Specific references

19. Austrian delegation data sheet, April 1996
20. Cardullo A.C., Ruszkowski A.M., De Leo V.A., J. Am. Acad. Dermatol., 21, 1989
21. Fong C.H., Hasegawa S. et al., Biosynthesis of Limonoid glucosides in lemon, J.Sci. Food Agric., 54, 393-398, 1991
22. Hagers, Handbuch der Pharmazeutischen Praxis, Springer-Verlag, Auflage, 4. Bd., Chemikalien und Drogen CI-G, 93-96, 1973
23. Nater J.P., De Groot A.C., Unwanted Effects of cosmetic and drugs used in Dermatology, Excerpta Medica, 315, 318, 1983
24. Melendreras F.A., Laencina J. et al., Aceites esenciales de frutos de variedades de limonero, Rev. Agroquim. Tecnol. Aliment., 25, 1, 133-143, 1985
25. Wagner H., Bladt S., Zgainski E.M., Drogenanalyse, Dunnschichtchromatographische Analyse von Arzneidrogen, Springer- Verlag, 188, 1983 - DAB 6

26. Ph Helv VII
27. Recommendations concerning undesirable active principles, 3.16, 28th meeting Committee of Experts on Cosmetic Products, Rome, 3-7 November 1997, Council of Europe

Citrus limon (L.) Burm (peel)

Botanical name[1]	*Citrus limon* (L.) Burm.
Botanical synonyms[2, 18]	*Citrus medica* L. ssp. *limonum* Hook f., *Citrus medica* L. ssp. *limonum* (Risso) Wight et Arn., C. *limonum* Risso
Botanical family	Rutaceae
Common names	Lemon (English)
	Zitroen (Dutch)
	Citron (French)
	Zitrone (German)
	Limone (Italian)
	Sitron (Norwegian)
	Limón (Spanish)
	Citron (Swedish)
EU INCI name[3]	*Citrus limonum*
CTFA INCI name[4]	Lemon (*Citrus medica limonum*) oil

CAS number	8008-56-8
EINECS number	-
Parts used	Peel

Important constituents including active principles[11]

Essential oil (0.2-0.6%)(17):
- Monoterpenes (up to 90%)[(11)] (d-limonene (up to 70%)[11], α- and β-pinene, β-phellandrene, camphene, sabinene, myrcene, cadinene, α- and β-terpinene, p-cymene, terpinolene, geraniol, terpinen-4-ol, linalool, citronellol, α- and β-terpineol, linalyl- and geranylacetate, geranial, neral, citronellal)
- Sesquiternenes (β-caryophyllene, α- and β-bisabolene, α-bergamotene)
- Coumarins (0.41-0.87%)[11] (bergamottin, bergapten, bergaferone, citropten, imperatorin, isoimperatorin, isopimpinellin, phellopterin, byakangelicin, byakangelicol, cnidicin, aurapten, umbelliferone, scopoletin, ossipeucedanin, 7-methoxy-5-geranoxycoumarin, 8-geranoxypsoralen)
- Alcohols (eptyl-,octyl-, nonyl-, decyl-, lauryl- and sinapyl alcohol) as acetate and propionate
- Aldehydes (2-6%)[11] (hexanal, eptanal, octanal, nonanal, decanal, undecanal and dodecanal)
- Organic acids (acetic, caprylic and lauric acid)
- Ketons (methyleptenon)

Preparation[29]	1) Lemon oil
	2) Terpeneless lemon oil

Manufacturing process[29]

1) Mechanical treatment of the fresh peels without heat
2) Concentration of the essential oil under reduced pressure or by solvent partition

Examples of specifications[29]

1) Relative density: 0.850 to 0.858
   Refractive index: 1.474 to 1.476
   Specific optical rotation: +57° to +70°
   Residue on evaporation: 1.8 to 3.6%
   Assay: 2.2 to 4.5% carbonyl compounds as citral
2) Relative density: 0.880 to 0.895
   Refractive index: 1.475 to 1.485
   Specific optical rotation: -5° to +2°
   Solubility in ethanol: soluble at 20° C, in 1 volume of ethanol 80% v/v
   Assay: not less than 40% aldehydes as citral

Intended cosmetic effects and used concentration in cosmetic products

Tonic, stimulant, refreshing, purifying, deodorant, insect repellent; fragrance

Up to 0.4% in detergents, creams and lotions

Other possible effects

Healing, anti-rheumatic and anti-nevralgic, in psoriasis treatment (by topical application), anti-microbial, rubefacient

Main toxicological data[24]

LD_{50} oral in rats: > 5000 mg/kg
LD_{50} dermal on rabbits: > 5000 mg/kg
Skin irritation on rabbits: moderately irritating
Skin irritation on human (25 subjects, after a 48-hour closed-patch test): no irritation
Sensitisation: no sensitisation reactions
Phototoxicity: distinct phototoxic effects

(d-limonene) [RTECS]
Carcinogenicity: tumourigenic (equivocal tumourigenic agent)

Databases used

CA Search 1967-95, Medline 1966-96, Embase 1974-95, Ref. Tox. Eff. Chem. Sub., Toxline, IPA, Napralert, Cosmet Database, HSDB

Keywords

Citrus limon

Evaluation and remarks

Cat. C (essential oil; terpeneless essential oil)

While the use of lemon oil poses problems for certain sensitive subjects on account of its allergenic limonene and citral content, the terpeneless essential oil, which contains no limonene carbides, still contains citral.

General references

1. Index Kewensis, Clarendon Press
2. Penso G., Index Plantarum Medicinalium Totius Mundi Eorumque Synonymorum, OEMF, 1983

3. European Commission Decision 96/335/EC of 8 May 1996, Official Journal of the European Community No. L132 of 1 June 1996

4. International Cosmetic Ingredient Dictionary 6th ed. CTFA, 1, 1995

5. Benigni R., Capra C., Cattorini P.E., Piante Medicinali chimica farmacologia e terapia, Inverni & Della Beffa, 2, 1, 828-839, 1964

6. Council of Europe, Flavouring Substances and natural sources of flavourings 3rd ed., Maisonneuve, (139, N1), 1981

7. Flavouring Extract Manufactures Association (Fema), Survey of flavouring ingredients usage levels, (No. 2625, 2626) Food Technology, 178 (280),

8. Fenaroli G., Sostanze Aromatiche Naturali, Hoepli ed., 696-704, 1963

9. Grieve M., A modern herbal, Barnes & Noble Books, 474-476, 1996

10. Guenther E., The essential oils, D. Van Nostrand, 3, 81- 115, 1958

11. Leung A.Y., Foster S., Encyclopedia of common natural ingredients, Wiley & Son Publ., 342-344,1995

12. Martindale 31st ed., The Royal Pharmaceutical Society, 1996

13. Merck Index 12th ed., Merck & Co. Inc., 1996

14. Paris R.R., Moyse H., Matière Médicale 2nd ed., Masson, 2, 300, 1981

15. Proserpio G., Martelli A., Patri G.F., Elementi di fitocosmesi, Sepem, 2, 669-670, 1983

16. Van Hellemont J., Compendium de Phytotherapie, APB, 104-106, 1986

17. Wichtl M., Teedrogen, WVG, 538-539, 1989

Specific references

18. Austrian delegation data sheet, April 1996

19. Yamamoto A., Kang S., Dosui K., Antioxidants from olive extracts for food, cosmetic and pharmaceutical preparations, JP 09 78,061 [97 78,061], 25 March 1997

20. Cardullo A.C. et al., Allergic contact dermatitis resulting from sensitivity to citrus peel, geraniol and citral, Journal of the American Academy of Dermatology, 21, 2,2, 395-397, 1989

21. Chamblee T.S., Clark B.C., Brewster G.B., Radford T., Iacobucci G.A., J. Agric. Food Chem., 39, 162-169, 1991

22. Lawrence B.M., Reynolds R.J., Progress in essential oil, Perfum. Flav., 14, 41-56, 1989

23. Nater J.P., De Groot A.C., Unwanted Effects of cosmetic and drugs used in Dermatology, Excerpta Medica, 315, 318, 1983

24. Opdyke. D.L.J., Food and Cosmetics Toxicology, 12, 5-6, 725-726, 1974

25. Opdyke. D.L.J., Food and Cosmetics Toxicology,1, 807, 1978

26. Stanley W.L. and Jurd L., Citrus coumarins, J. Agr. Food Chem. 19, 6, 1106-1110, 1971

27. Ziegler H., Spiteller G., Coumarins and Psoralens from Sicilian Lemon oil , Flavour Fragr. J., 7, 129-139, 1992
28. Ziegler H., Spiteller G., Identification of sinapyl alcohol derivatives in sicilian lemon oil, J. Essent. Oil Res., 4, 355-361, 1992
29. BP '93
30. FU IX

Citrus sinensis (L.) Osbeck (fresh flowers)

Botanical name[1]	*Citrus sinensis* (L.) Osbeck
Botanical synonyms[2, 13, 20]	*Citrus aurantium* L. ssp. amara (L.) Engl., *Citrus vulgaris* Risso, *Citrus bigaradia* Risso, *Citrus amara* Link
Botanical family	Rutaceae
Common names	Orange (English)
	Oranje (Dutch)
	Orange (French)
	Orange (German)
	Arancia (Italian)
	Bitterapplsin (Norwegian)
	Naranja (Spanish)
	Apelsin (Swedish)
EU INCI name[3]	*Citrus amara*
CTFA INCI name[4]	Bitter orange (*Citrus aurantium amara*) oil

CAS number	72968-50-4 (orange sour extract)
	84012-28-2
EINECS number	277-143-2 (orange sour extract)
Parts used	Fresh flowers

Important constituents including active principles[12]

Essential oil: up to 0.12%:

– Monoterpenes (limonene 15%, dipentene, α- and β-pinene 11%, camphene, linalool (30-60%)[16] and linalyl acetate (6-17%)[16], nerol and neryl acetate, geraniol, nerolidol 6%, a-terpineol, citral)
– Sesquiterpenes (farnesol)
– Aldehydes (nonanal, decanal, dodecanal)
– Ketone (Jasmone)
– Phenylethylalcohol
– Indole
– Methyl anthranilate (0.5-1.2%)[10]
– Organic acids (acetic, phenyl acetic and benzoic) in ester form
– Paraffins
– Other compounds (in traces): cis-8-heptadecene, 2,5-dimethyl-2-vinyl-4-hexenal, valeric acid

Preparation

1) Essential oil (*Aurantii floris aetheroleum*)[28] or Neroli
2) Distilled water

Manufacturing process

1) Steam distillation
2) Water collected from steam distillate W/D = 1:1

Examples of specifications

1)[28.] Relative density: 0.870 to 0.883
Specific optical rotation: +1.5° to +12°
Refractive index: 1.468 to 1.474
Solubility in ethanol: soluble at 20°, in 2 parts of ethanol 80% v/v

Intended cosmetic effects and used concentration in cosmetic products

(essential oil)
Tonic, stimulant, dermopurifying; fragrance; flavour
Concentration limited in preparations for impure and greasy skin, massage lotions

Up to 1% in fragrances

(distilled water)
Tonic, refreshing, soothing; fragrance

Up to 50% in solutions, gels and lotions for eye contour, delicate and sensitive skin

Other possible effects

Antimicrobial, anti-inflammatory

Neroli bigarade oil was 5.5 times more effective as a bactericidal agentthan pheno[24.]

Main toxicological data[24.]

LD_{50} oral in rats: 4.55 + 0.105 g/kg
LD_{50} dermal on rabbits: > 5 g/kg
Irritation in rabbits: hairless mice and swine: no irritation
Irritation in humans: no irritation after 48-hour closed-patch test
Sensitisation in humans (25 volunteers): no sensitisation reactions
Phototoxicity in hairless mice and swine: no phototoxic effects were reported

Databases used

CA Search 1967-95, Medline 1966-96, Embase 1974-95,
Ref. Tox. Eff. Chem. Sub., Toxline, IPA, Napralert, Cosmet Database

Keywords

Citrus sinensis

Evaluation and remarks

Cat. A (essential oil or neroli; distilled water)

On account of the presence of monoterpenes, Citrus essential oils should be specially labelled.
Nonetheless, no toxic effects are reported.
Distilled water would in any case be even less toxic.

General references

1. Index Kewensis, Clarendon Press
2. Penso G., Index Plantarum Medicinalium Totius Mundi Eorumque Synonymorum, OEMF, 1983
3. European Commission Decision 96/335/EC of 8 May 1996, Official Journal of the European Community No. L132 of 1 June 1996
4. International Cosmetic Ingredient Dictionary 6th ed. CTFA, 1,1995
5. Comprehensive Licensing Standards of Cosmetics by Category, 1, 193, Yakuji Nippo Ltd., 1986

6. Comprehensive Licensing Standards of Cosmetics by Category, 4 313, Yakuji Nippo Ltd., 1989
7. Council of Europe, Flavouring Substances and natural sources of flavourings 3rd ed., (136, N2/143,N2), Maisonneuve, 1981
8. Flavouring Extract Manufactures Association (Fema), Survey of flavouring ingredients usage levels, (No. 2819, 2821), Food Technology, 185 (287), 1965
9. Grieve M., A modern herbal, Barnes & Noble Books, 601-602,1996
10. Guenther E., The essential oils, D. Van Nostrand, 3, 228- 260, 1958
11. Japanese Cosmetic Ingredients Codex, Yakuji Nippo LTD., 536, 1993
12. Leung A.Y., Foster S, Encyclopedia of common natural ingredients, Wiley & Son Publ., 393-397,1995
13. Merck Index 12th ed., Merck & Co. Inc., 1996
14. Monographs Aurantii flos/ Aurantii floris aetheroleum, Bundesanzeiger, No. 128 (Jul.14,1993), through Le monografie tedesche, Studio Edizioni, 3, 1995
15. Paris R.R., Moyse H., Matière Médicale 2nd ed., Masson, 2, 297-298, 1981
16. Proserpio G., Martelli A., Patri G.F., Elementi di fitocosmesi, Sepem, 2, 664-665, 1983
17. Van Hellemont J., Compendium de Phytotherapie, APB, 104-106, 1986
18. Wichtl M., Teedrogen, WVG, 357-358, 377-378, 1989

Specific references

19. Austian delegation data sheet, April 1996
20. Dubery I.A. and Schabort J., Calmodulin from Citrus sinensis: purification and characterisation, Phytochemistry, 26, 1, 37-40, 1987
21. Hagers, Handbuch der Pharmazeutischen Praxis, Springer-Verlag, 4. Auflage, 4. Bd., Chemikalien und Drogen CI-G, 90-93, 1973
22. Nordby H.E. and Nagy S., Fatty acid composition of sterol esters from Citrus sinensis, Citrus paradisi, Citrus limon aurantifolia and Citrus limettioides Sac, Phytochemistry, 13, 443-452, 1974
23. Olumide Y., Contact Dermatitis, 17, 85-88, 1987
24. Opdyke. D.L.J., Food and Cosmetics Toxicology, 14, 813-814, 1976
25. Peleg H. et al., Distribution of bound and free phenolic acid in oranges (Citrus sinensis) and grapefruits (Citrus paradisi), J. Sci. Food Agric. 57, 417-426, 1991
26. Volden G., Krokan H., Kavli G., Midelfart K., Contact Dermatitis, 9, 201-1983
27. Ziegler G. and Spiteller G., A coumarin and a diterpene from Citrus sinensis (L.) Osbeck cv Valencia (Rutaceae), Flavour and Fragrance Journal, 7, 141-145, 1992
28. Ph Helv VII

29. DAB 9
30. Erg B 6
31. FU IX
32. OAB '83
33. Ph Helv VII

Citrus sinensis (L.) Osbeck (fruits)

Botanical name[1]	*Citrus sinensis* (L.) Osbeck
Botanical synonyms[1, 15]	*Citrus aurantium* L. var. *sinensis*, *Citrus sinensis* (L.) Pers., *Citrus aurantium* ssp. *Sinensis* Engl.
Botanical family	Rutaceae
Common names	Orange (English)
	Oranje (Dutch)
	Orange (French)
	Orange (German)
	Arancia (Italian)
	Bitterappelsin (Norwegian)
	Naranja dulce (Spanish)
	Apelsin (Swedish)
EU INCI name[3]	*Citrus dulcis*
CTFA INCI name[4]	Orange (*Citrus aurantium dulcis*) extract

CAS number	8028-48-6 (orange sweet extract)
	84012-28-2
EINECS number	232-433-8 (orange sweet extract)
Parts used	Fruits

Important constituents including active principles[12]

- Essential oil: (see monograph)
- Flavonoids (neohesperidin, hesperidin, narirutin, auranetin, tangeretin, kaempferol, nobiletin, sinensetin)
- Diterpenes (gomerol, 6, 7-dimethoxycoumarin)[25]
- Vitamins (A, B group, C (0.03-0.08%) and E)
- Triterpenoid: bitter principle (limonin)
- Coumarins (auraptene)[25]
- Phytosterols and their esters[22]
- Phenol acids (hydroxycinnamic, ferulic, sinapic, coumaric, caffeic acid)[24]
- Organic acids (malic, citric acid) (0.9-3%)[15]
- Proteins (mainly calmodulin)[20]
- Carotenoids
- Pectins
- Citrantin
- Sugars (1-8%)[15]

Preparation	1) Orange extract (2)[7]
	2) Orange extract[6]
Manufacturing process	1)[7] Extraction with propylene glycol
	2)[6] Compression of the fruits and sometimes addition of concentrated glycerin
Examples of specifications	1)[7] Heavy metals: not more than 20 ppm
	Arsenic: not more than 2 ppm
	2)[6] Heavy metals: not more than 20 ppm
	Arsenic: not more than 2 ppm

Intended cosmetic effects and used concentration in cosmetic products

Tonic, protective, refreshing, moisturising, dermopurifying; fragrance; flavour

Concentration limited in preparations for impure, sensitive and ageing skin

Other possible effects

Anti-inflammatory, microvessels protectant, free radical scavenger (flavonoids). Cheratolitic. Antimicrobial.

Main toxicological data

LD_{50} oral in rats > 5 g/kg

LD_{50} dermal on rats: > 5 g/kg

Skin irritation on rabbits: moderately irritating

Subchronic oral toxicity in rats (male, 13 weeks): 5 mg/kg

Mutagenicity in Chinese Hamster Chromosome Abberations: negative

Carcinogenicity studies in mice: tumorigenic, neoplastic gastro-intestinal tumours.

Databases used

CA Search 1967-95, Medline 1966-96, Embase 1974-95,
Ref. Tox. Eff. Chem. Sub., Toxline, IPA, Napralert, Cosmet database

Keywords

Citrus sinensis

Evaluation and remarks

Cat. A (propylene glycol extract; extract by compression)

***A priori*, the quantity of essential oil and coumarins in the preparations should be very small, removing any risk of toxicity.**

General references

1. Index Kewensis, Clarendon Press
2. Penso G., Index Plantarum Medicinalium Totius Mundi Eorumque Synonymorum, OEMF, 1983
3. European Commission Decision 96/335/EC of 8 May 1996, Official Journal of the European Community No. L132 of 1 June 1996
4. International Cosmetic Ingredient Dictionary 6th ed. CTFA, *1*, 1995
5. Benigni R., Capra C., Cattorini P.E., Piante Medicinali chimica farmacologia e terapia, Inverni & Della Beffa, *1*, 98-100, 1971
6. Comprehensive Licensing Standards of Cosmetics by Category, *1*, 193, 1986

7. Comprehensive Licensing Standards of Cosmetics by Category, 4 313, 1989
8. Council of Europe, Flavouring Substances and natural sources of flavourings 3rd ed., (136 N2;143 N2), Maisonneuve, 1981
9. Flavouring Extract Manufactures Association (Fema), Survey of flavouring ingredients usage levels, (No. 2825), Food Technology, 186 (288), 1965
10. Grieve M., A modern herbal, Barnes & Noble Books, 2, 601-602,1996
11. Japanese Cosmetic Ingredients Codex, Yakuji Nippo LTD., 535-536, 1993
12. Leung A.Y:, Foster S, Encyclopedia of common natural ingredients, Wiley & Son Publ., 393-397,1995
13. Merck Index 12th ed., Merck & Co. Inc., 1996
14. Monographs Citri sinensis pericarpium, Bundesanzeiger, No. 22a (Febr. 01,1990), through Le monografie tedesche, Studio Edizioni, 1, 1994
15. Paris R.R., Moyse H., Matière Médicale 2nd ed., Masson, 2, 298, 1981
16. Proserpio G., Martelli A., Patri G.F., Elementi di fitocosmesi, Sepem, 2, 666, 1983
17. Van Hellemont J., Compendium de Phytotherapie, APB, 104-106, 1986
18. Wichtl M., Teedrogen, WVG, 357-358, 377-378, 1989

Specific references

19. Austian delegation data sheet, April 1996
20. Dubery I.A. and Schabort J.C., Calmodulin from Citrus sinensis: purification and characterisation, Phytochemistry, 26, 1, 37-40, 1987
21. Hagers, Handbuch der Pharmazeutischen Praxis, Springer-Verlag, Auflage, 4. Bd., Chemikalien und Drogen CI-G, 90-93, 1973
22. Nordby H.E. and Nagy S., Fatty acid composition of sterol esters from Citrus sinensis, Citrus paradisi, Citrus limon aurantifolia and Citrus limettioides sacs, Phytochemistry, 13, 443-452, 1974
23. Olumide Y., Contact Dermatitis, 17, 85-88, 1987
24. Peleg H. et al. Distribution of bound and free Phenolic acids in oranges (Citrus sinensis) and grapefruits (Citrus paradisi), J. Sci. Food Agric. 57, 417-426, 1991
25. Ziegler G. and Spitteler G., A coumarin and Diterpene from Citrus sinensis (L.) Osbeck cv. Valencia (Rutaceae), Flavour and Fragrance Journal 7, 141-145, 1992
26. Volden G., Krokan H., Kavli G., Midelfart K., Contact Dermatitis, 9, 201- 204, 1983
27. DAB 9
28. Erg B 6
29. FU IX
30. OAB '83
31. Ph Helv VII

Citrus sinensis (L.) Osbeck (fresh peel)

Botanical name[1]	*Citrus sinensis* (L.) Osbeck
Botanical synonyms[2]	*Citrus aurantium* L. var. *Sinensis*, *Citrus sinensis* (L.) Pers., *Citrus aurantium* ssp. *sinensis* Engl.
Botanical family	Rutaceae
Common names	Orange (English)
	Oranje (Dutch)
	Orange (French)
	Orange (German)
	Arancia (Italian)
	Bitterappelsin (Norwegian)
	Naranja dulce (Spanish)
	Apelsin (Swedish)
EU INCI name[3]	*Citrus dulcis*
CTFA INCI name[4]	Orange (*Citrus aurantium dulcis*) oil

CAS number	8028-48-6 (orange sweet extract)
	8008-57-9
EINECS number	232-433-8 (orange sweet extract)
Parts used	Fresh peels

Important constituents including active principles[11]

1) Essential oil (up to 2.5%)[11]:

Monoterpenes (d limonene (up to 90%)[11], α-terpinene, linalool, linalyl acetate, geraniol, geranyl acetate, nerol, α-terpineol, citronellol, citral, citronellal)

– Sesquiterpenes (farnesol, nookatene[20], valencene[20], α-ylangene[11])
– Alcohols (nonylalcohol)
– Aldehydes (1.2-2.5%)[11] (octanal, nona, decanal and dodecanal)
– Acetaldehydes (trans-2-hexenal)
– Esters (methyl-anthranylate, ethyl-butyrate)
– Coumarins (bergaptene, auraptenol)
– Organic acid (octadecadienoic acid)

Preparation[24]	1) Essential oil (*Orange oil*)
	2) Essential oil terpeneless (*Terpeneless orange oil*)
Manufacturing process[24]	1) Expression by mechanical means from the fresh peels
	2) Concentration under reduced pressure or by solvent partition

Examples of specifications[24]
   1) Relative density: 0.842 to 0.848
   Refractive index: 1.472 to 1.476
   Specific optical rotation: +94° to +99 °
   Residue on evaporation: 1.0 to 5.0
   Solubility in ethanol: soluble at 20°, in 7 parts of ethanol 90%
   Content of aldehydes: not less than 1% w/w as decanal
   2) Relative density: 0.855 to 0.880
   Refractive index: 1.461 to 1.473
   Specific optical rotation: not more than + 60°
   Solubility in ethanol: soluble at 20°, in 1 part of ethanol 90%
   Content of aldehydes: not less than 18% w/w as decanal

Intended cosmetic effects and used concentration in cosmetic products
   Tonic, purifying, lightening; fragrance, flavour
   In preparations for delicate and sensitive skin (masks)
   Up to 0.4% in soaps, emulsions, gels and solutions

Other possible effects
   Antimicrobial, anti-inflammatory[11], whitening

Main toxicological data[22]
   LD_{50} oral in rats: > 5 000 mg/kg
   LD50 dermal in rats: > 5 000 mg/kg
   Skin irritation in mice: not irritating
   Skin irritation in rabbits: moderately irritating
   Irritation in humans (21volunteers): after 48-hour closed-patch test
   8% in petrolatum produced no sensitisation reactions
   Phototoxicity: no phototoxic effects were reported
   Subchronic oral toxicity in rats (male, 13 weeks): 5 mg/kg
   Mutagenicity in Chinese Hamster Chromosome Aberrations: negative
   Carcinogenicity in mice: tumorigenic, neoplastic gastrointestinal tumours

   Note: Contact dermatitis by orange oil was pointed out[21]

Databases used
   CA Search 1967-95, Medline 1966-96, Embase 1974-95,
   Ref. Tox. Eff. Chem. Sub., Toxline, IPA, Napralert, Cosmet

Keywords
   Citrus sinensis

Evaluation and remarks
   Group: A (When deterpeneless and without psoralenes)

General references
   1. Index Kewensis, Clarendon Press
   2. Penso G., Index Plantarum Medicinalium Totius Mundi Eorumque Synonymorum, OEMF, 1983
   3. European Commission Decision 96/335/EC of 8 May 1996, Official Journal of the European Community No. L132 of 1 June 1996
   4. International Cosmetic Ingredient Dictionary 6th ed. CTFA, *1*, 1995
   5. Benigni R., Capra C., Cattorini P.E., Piante Medicinali chimica farmacologia e terapia, Inverni & Della Beffa, *1*, 98-100, 1971
   6. Council of Europe, Flavouring Substances and natural sources of flavourings 3rd ed., (136, N2/143,N2), Maisonneuve, 1981

7. Flavouring Extract Manufactures Association (Fema), Survey of flavouring ingredients usage levels, (No. 2822, 2825, 2826), Food Technology, 186 (288), 1965

8. Fenaroli G., Sostanze Aromatiche Naturali, Hoepli ed., 344-357,1963

9. Grieve M., A modern herbal, Barnes & Noble Books, 2, 601-602,1996

10. Guenther E., The essential oils, D. Van Nostrand, 3, 118- 197, 1958

11. Leung A.Y:, Foster S, Encyclopedia of common natural ingredients, Wiley & Son Publ., 393-397,1995

12. Martindale 31st ed., The Royal Pharmaceutical Society, 1996

13. Merck Index 12th ed., Merck & Co. Inc., 1996

14. Paris R.R., Moyse H., Matière Médicale 2nd ed., Masson, 2, 298, 1981

15. Proserpio G., Martelli A., Patri G.F., Elementi di fitocosmesi, Sepem, 2, 666, 1983

16. Van Hellemont J., Compendium de Phytotherapie, APB, 104-106, 1986

Specific references

17. Dugo G et al., On the genuineness of Citrus Essential oil. Part XLIII: the composition of the volatile fraction of Italian sweet orange oils (*Citrus sinensis* (L.) Osbeck), J. Essent.Oil Res. 6, 101-137, 1994

18. Hagers, Handbuch der Pharmazeutischen Praxis, Springer-Verlag, 4. Auflage, 4. Bd., Chemikalien und Drogen CI-G, 90-93, 1973

19. Karawya M.S., Balbaa S.I. and Hifnawy M.S., Peel oils of different types of *Citrus sinensis* L. and *Citrus aurantium* L. growing in Egypt, Journal of Pharmaceutical Sciences, 60, 3, 381-386, 1971

20. Lund E.D., Coleman L. and Moshonas M.G., Nootkatene from *Citrus sinensis,* Phytochemistry, 9, 2419-2422, 1970

21. Olumide Y., Contact Dermatitis in Nigeria (I). Hand dermatitis in women, Contact Dermatitis, 17, 85-88, 1987

22. Opdyke. D.L.J., Food and Cosmetics Toxicology, 12, 733-734, 1974

23. Volden G., Krokan H., Kavli G., Midelfart K., Phototoxic and contact toxic reactions of the exocarp of sweet oranges: a common cause of chelitis?, Contact Dermatitis, 9, 201-204, 1983

24. BP '93

25. - Ph Helv. VII

26. - FU IX

Commiphora myrrha

Botanical name[1]	*Commiphora myrrha* Engl. var. *molmol* and *Commiphora abyssinica* Engl.
Botanical synonyms[2] **of** *Commiphora myrrha*	
	Balsamea myrrha Baill., *Balsamodendron myrrha* Ness.
Botanical family	Burseraceae
Common names	Myrrh (English)
	Mirre (Dutch)
	Mirhami (Finnish)
	Myrrhe (French)
	Myrrhe (German)
	Mirra (Italian)
	Myrra (Norwegian)
	Mirra (Spanish)
	Myrra (Swedish)
EU INCI name[3]	*Commiphora myrrha*
CTFA INCI name[4]	Myrrh (*Commiphora myrrha*)
	Myrrh (*Commiphora myrrha*) extract
	Myrrh (*Commiphora myrrha*) oil

CAS number	84929-26-0 100084-96-6 (*Commiphora myrrha*)
	8016-37-3 (*Myrrh absolute*)
	9000-45-7 (*Commiphora abyssinica*)
EINECS number	284-510-0 309-134-7 (*Commiphora myrrha*)
	232-543-6 (*Commiphora abyssinica*)
Parts used	Resin gum (myrrh)

Important constituents including active principles[9, 13]

– Resin gum:

(Essential oil (about 8%): Heerabolene, limonene, dipentene, pinene, eugenol, cinnamaldehyde, cuminaldehyde, cumic alcohol, cadinene, m-cresol, curzerenone, curzerene, dihydro-pyrocurzerenone, furanoeudesma-1,3-diene, 1,10-furanodiene-6-one and lindestrene (3.5%)

Resin (about 20%): α, β and γ-commiphoric acid, commiphorinic acid, α and β-heerabomyrrhols, heeraboresene, commiferin, campesterol, β-sitosterol, cholesterol, α-amyrone, 3-epi-α-amyrin

Gum (about 60%):

Polysaccharides: conteing arabinose, galactose, xylose and 4-0-

methylglucuronic acid (about 65%)
Furanosesquiterpenoids)
– Proteins (about 20%)
– Organic acids: (palmitic, formic and acetic acids)

Preparation

1) Essential oil
2) Tincture T/D = 5:1
3) Absolute myrrh (a resinous mass)

Manufacturing process

1) Extraction from the crushed gum by steam distillation[8.]
2) Maceration of resin gum with alcohol 90%
3) Extraction of myrrh resinoid with absolute alcohol

Examples of specifications

1)[8.] Specific gravity at 15°/15°: 0.995 to 1.010
Specific optical rotation: – 62° 32' to – 83° 55'
Refractive index at 20°: 1.5211 to 1.5241
Acid number: 2.0 to 3.7
Saponification number: 16.0 to 35.5
Solubility: soluble in 7.5 to 8.5 and more vol. of alcohol 90%
2) Dry residue: not less than 4%

Intended cosmetic effects and used concentration in cosmetic products

Astringent, tonic; purifying

(resin gum)
Up to 10% in toothpastes, mouthwashes as soothing agent, products for nail protection

(essential oil)
Up to 0.8% in fragrances as fixative

Other possible effects

Stimulant, antiseptic, deodorising for fresh breath; granulation-promoting agent[16.]

Main toxicological data

(Essential oil)[18.]:
LD_{50} oral in rats: 1650 mg/kg
Primary skin irritation: 1% myrrh oil in methanol and undiluted myrrh oil was not irritating to hairless mice and swine. No irritation was reported from 8% myrrh oil in petrolatum in 48-hour patch-test on human volunteers
Sensitisation: no reaction reported in volunteers treated with 8% myrrh in petrolatum
Phototoxicity: 1% myrrh in methanol was not phototoxic to hairless mice.

(Myrrh absolute)[19.]:
Irritation: after open-patch application to hairless mice and miniature swine. A 1% solution in methanol is not irritating. A 48-hour closed-patch test with 8% in petrolatum on the backs or forearms of 53 volunteers produced no irritation.
Sensitisation: a 22-year-old patient who developed contact dermatitis to benzoin tincture followed by non-eczematous exanthem was given 18 closed-patch tests with various gum. A cross-sensitisation reaction was produced by myrrh gum (concentration and vehicle unknown). Maximisation tests were carried out with 8% in

petrolatum on 53 volunteers in two separate panels using two different samples: sample 75-103 produced 2/25 sensitisation reactions; sample 80-89 produced 0/28 reactions. This test concentration was based on a reported maximum concentration of 0.8% in consumer products.

Phototoxicity: no phototoxicity effects were produced when 1% in methanol was applied to the skin of hairless mice or miniature swine, followed by UVA irradiation with blacklight or xenon lamp.

Databases used	CA Search 1967-96, Medline 1966-96, Embase 1974-95, Ref. Tox. Eff. Chem. Sub., Toxline, Biosis, HDSB.
Keywords	*Commiphora abyssinica, Arabian myrrh, Commiphora myrrha*
Evaluation and remarks	**Cat. A**

General references

1. Index Kewensis, Clarendon Press
2. Penso G., Index Plantarum Medicinalium Totius Mundi Eorumque Synonymorum, OEMF, 1983
3. European Commission Decision 96/335/EC of 8 May 1996, Official Journal of the European Community No. L132 of 1 June 1996
4. International Cosmetic Ingredient Dictionary 6th ed., CTFA, *1*, 1995
5. Council of Europe, Flavouring substances and natural sources of flavourings 3rd ed., Maisonneuve, (150, N2), 1981
6. Fenaroli G., Sostanze Aromatiche Naturali, Hoepli ed., 763-765, 1963
7. Flavouring Extract Manufactures Association (Fema), Survey of flavouring ingredients usage levels, (No. 2765, 2766) Food Technology, (285), 1965
8. Guenther E., The essential oils, D. Van Nostrand, *4*, 344-348, 1952
9. Leung A.Y., Foster S., Encyclopedia of common natural ingredients, Wiley & Son Publ., 382-383, 1996
10. Martindale 31st ed., The Royal Pharmaceutical Society, 1996
11. Merck Index 12th ed., Merck & Co. Inc., 1996
12. Monographs Myrrha, Bundesanzeiger, No. 193, (Oct. 15, 1987), through Le monografie tedesche, Studio Edizioni, *2*, 1994
13. Newall C., Anderson L., Phillipson J.D., Herbal Medicines: a guide for health care professionals, The Pharmaceutical Press, 199-200, 1996
14. Proserpio G., Martelli A., Patri G.F., Elementi di fitocosmesi, Sepem, *2*, 671, 1982
15. Wichtl M., Teedrogen, WVG, 349-351, 1989

Specific references

16. Delaveau P., Lallouette P., Tessier A.M., Drogues Végétales Stimulant l'Activité Phagocytaire du Système Réticulo-Endothélial, Planta Medica, *40*, 49-54,1980
17. Nardi U., L'impiego della mirra nella cosmesi ungueale, E.D., *11*, 60-2, 1993

18. Opdyke D., Food and Cosmetics Toxicology, *14*, 621, 1976
19. Opdyke D., Food and Chemical Toxicology, *30*, 91S, 1992
20. OAB '83
21. DAB 9
22. Ph. Helv. VII
23. Br. Herb. Ph. '90

Cupressus sempervirens

Botanical name[1]	*Cupressus sempervirens* L.
Botanical synonyms[1]	*Cupressus fastigiata* D.C.
Botanical family	Cupressaceae

Common names		
	Cypress	(English)
	Cypres	(Dutch)
	Sypressi	(Finnish)
	Cyprès commun	(French)
	Echte Zypresse	(German)
	Cipresso	(Italian)
	Sypress	(Norwegian)
	Ciprés común	(Spanish)
	Cypress	(Swedish)

EU INCI name[2]	*Cupressus sempervirens*
CTFA INCI names[3]	Cypress (*Cupressus sempervirens*) extract Cypress (*Cupressus sempervirens*) oil

CAS number	84696-07-1 8013-86-3 (essential oil)
EINECS number	283-626-9
Parts used	Leaves and branches, dried fruits (cones)

Important constituents including active principles[5, 7, 10, 12]

- Essential oil (up to 1%)[10]:
  (Monoterpenes: α and β-pinene, camphene, sabinene, δ^3-carene, myrcene, α-terpinene, limonene, cineole, β-ocimene, γ-terpinene, π-cymene, terpinolene, karahanaenone, linalool, karahanaenol, bornyl acetate, terpinene acetate, α-terpineol, borneol, π-cymenol Sesquiterpenes: α and β-cedrene, thuyopsene, δ and ϵ-cadinene, α-cadinol, α-cubebene, cedrol or "cypress camphor" Diterpenes: sandaracopimaradiene, manoyl oxide, biformine, dehydroabietane; diterpene acids: neocupressic acid I, II, III, IV11. Phenol acids: carvacrol)

- Polyphenols
  (Dimeric flavonoids: amentoflavone, cupressoflavone Procyanidols and cathechins[15]
  Cathechic tannins (3-5%)[10]

Preparation	1) Essential oil 2) Hydroglycolic extract E/D = 5:1[13]

Manufacturing process	1) Steam distillation of leaves and branches[7]
	2) Percolation of fruits with propylene glycol 50%

Examples of specifications 1)[7] Specific gravity at 15°/15°: 0.870 to 0.891
Specific optical rotation: +4° 32' to +29° 20'
Refractive index: 1.4740 to 1.4821
Saponification number: 5.1 to 19.6
Solubility in 5.5 to 10 vol. of 90% alcohol. Sometimes turbid in 10 vol

2)[13] pH: 5.5 to 6.5
Relative density at 20°: 1.037 to 1.043
Refractive index at 20°: 1.388 to 1.394
Dry residue: 0.20 to 1.00%
Heavy metals: ≤ 5 ppm

Intended cosmetic effects and used concentration in cosmetic products

Astringent, skin protectant, purifying; fragrance

(essential oil)
Up to 0.1% in soaps and detergents

(glycolic extract)
up to 10% in creams, lotions and gels for couperosic skin, pre- and after- sun products, deodorants

Other possible effects Veinous astringent, haemostatic, granulation promoting agent, free-radical scavenger, antibacterial[14]

Main toxicological data[16] LD_{50} oral in rats: >5 000 mg/kg
LD_{50} dermal in rabbits: >5 000 mg/kg
Primary skin irration. Undiluted oil applied to the hairless mice and swine was not irritating. Applied undiluted to intact or abraded rabbit skin for 24 hours under occlusion it was moderately irritating. Tested at 5% in petrolatum, it produced no irritation after a 48-hour closed-patch test on human subjects.
Sensitisation. Tested at 5% in petrolatum it produced no sensitisation among 25 human volunteers.
Phototoxicity: no phototoxic effects were reported in hairless mice and swine.

(Eucalyptol or 1,8-cineole or p-cineole)
has been studied sub-chronically in rats and mice; a NOEL of 300 mg/kg bw has been established. Eucalyptol has been found non mutagenic in different systems[17]

Databases used CA Search 1967-96, Medline 1966-96, Embase 1974-96, Ref. Tox. Eff. Chem. Sub., Toxline, Biosis, HDSB

Keywords *Cupressus sempervirens,* Cypress

Evaluation and remarks Cat. A

General references 1. Index Kewensis, Clarendon Press

2. European Commission Decision 96/335/EC of 8 May 1996, Official Journal of the European Community No. L132 of 1 June 1996

3. International Cosmetic Ingredient Dictionary 6th ed., CTFA, 1,1995

4. Benigni R., Capra C., Cattorini P.E., Piante Medicinali chimica farmacologia e terapia, Inverni & Della Beffa, *1*, 322-323, 1971

5. Council of Europe, Flavouring substances and natural sources of flavourings 3rd ed., Maisonneuve, (162 N2), 1981

6. Fenaroli G., Sostanze Aromatiche Naturali, Hoepli ed., 490-494, 1963

7. Guenther E., The essential oils, D. Van Nostrand, *6*, 332-336, 1952

8. Martindale 31st ed., The Royal Pharmaceutical Society, 1996

9. Merck Index 12th ed., Merck & Co. Inc., 1996

10. Van Hellemont J., Compendium de Phytotherapie, APB, 124,1986

Specific references

11. Bernard P., Susplugas P.et al., Séparation Rapide des Acides Diterpéniques Contenus dans les Galbules de Cyprès, Cupressus sempervirens L., Au Moyen de la Chromatographie Liquide Préparative Plantes médicinales et phytothérapie, *12*, 2, 137-143, 1978

12. Garnero G., Buil P., Joulain D., Tabacchi R., Parf. Cosm. Aromes, 20, 1978

13. Indena Product Specification, 1996

14. Izzo A.A., Di Carlo G., De Fusco R. et al., Biologial Screening of Italian Medicinal Plants for Antibacterial Activity, Phyto therapy Research 9, 1995

15. Jonadet M., Meunier M.T., Villie F. et al., Catéchines et oligomèrs flavanoliques de *Cupressus sempervirens* L. Activités inhibitrices vis-à-vis de l'élastase in vitro et activités angioprotectrices comparées in vivo, Ann. pharmaceutiques françaises, *42*, 2, 161-167, 1984

16. Opdyke D.L.J., Food and Cosmetics Toxicology, 16S, 699, 1978

17. Recommendations concerning undesirable active principles, 3.8, 28th meeting Committee of Experts on Cosmetic Products, Rome, 3-7 November 1997, Council of Europe

Foeniculum vulgare

Botanical name[1]	*Foeniculum vulgare* Mill. var. *dulce* Mill. and *Foeniculum vulgare* Mill. var. *amara*
Botanical synonyms[2]	*Anethum foeniculum* L., *Foeniculum capillaceum* Gilib., *Foeniculum officinale* All., *Foeniculum vulgare* Mill. var. *vulgare* Thell.
Botanical family	Apiaceae
Common names	Fennel (English)
	Venkel (Dutch)
	Fenkoli (Finnish)
	Fenouil (French)
	Fenchel (German)
	Finocchio selvatico (Italian)
	Fennikel (Norwegian)
	Hinojo (Spanish)
	Fänkål (Swedish)
EU INCI name[3]	*Foeniculum vulgare*
CTFA INCI name[4]	Fennel (*Foeniculum vulgare*)
	Fennel (*Foeniculum vulgare*) extract
	Fennel (*Foeniculum vulgare*) oil

CAS number	84625-39-8 (extract)
	85085-33-2 (extract)
	8006-84-6 (essential oil)
EINECS number	283-414-6 (extract)
Parts used	Fruits and roots

Important constituents including active principles[5, 8, 20]

- Essential oil (4-6%):
  (Monoterpenes: α-pinene (1.8-4.8%)[20] and β-pinene, α- and β-thujene, camphene, limonene (1.5-2.5%)20., β-phellandrene, D3-carene, sabinene, myrcene, terpinene, π-cymene, terpinolene, fenchone (up to 22%))[13]
  Sesquiterpenes
  Aldehydes: anisaldehyde
  Phenol ethers: trans-anethol (50-90%)[13], estragole (5-20%)[19]
  Coumarins: bergapten, xanthotoxin, marmesin, 7-hydroxy-coumarin)
- Flavonoids (mainly quercetin-3-glucuronide, rutin, isoquercitrin, quercetin-3-arabinoside, kaempferol-3-glucuronide, kaempferol-3-arabinoside)

    – Triterpenes (α-amirin)
    – Triglycerides (9-28%)[13] (containing mainly petroselinic, oleic, linoleic acids)
    – Phytosterols (b-sitosterol, stigmasterol)
    – Pectins (3%)[5]
    – Proteins (14-22%)[5]
    – Vitamins (tocopherols)

Preparation

1) Essential oil
2) Fennel extract[6]
3) Fluid extract E/D = 1:1
4) Tincture T/D = 5:1

Manufacturing process

1) Steam distillation of the crushed fruits[8, 11]
2) Percolation with propylene glycol 50%[6]
3) Percolation with alcohol 70% and concentration under vacuum[5, 8]
4) Maceration with alcohol 70%5.

Examples of specifications

1)[11] Specific gravity at 15°/15°: 0.965 to 0.977
    Specific optical rotation at 25°: +11° 0' to +20° 0'
    Refractive index at 20°: 1.528 to 1.539
    Congealing point: +5° to +10°
    Solubility: soluble in 5 vol. of alcohol 80% and in 0.5 vol. of alcohol 90%
2)[6] Heavy metals: not more than 20 ppm
    Arsenic: not more than 2 ppm

Intended cosmetic effects and used concentration in cosmetic products

Tonic, soothing, purifying; fragrance
Up to 0.4% in emulsions and detergents in products for eye area and oral mucosae (traditional use)

Other possible effects

Stimulant, granulation-promoting agent., antibacterial

Main toxicological data

(Fennel)[23, 25, 27]
LD_{50} oral in rats: 3800 mg/kg[27]
LD_{50} dermal in rabbits: > 5000 mg/kg[27]

Skin irritation:[27]
(Fennel oil)
Undiluted is severely irritating to hairless mice.
Applied for 24-hours under occlusion to intact or abraded rabbit skin is moderately irritating.
Diluted 4% in petrolatum is not irritating to human volunteers in 48-hour closed-patch tests.
Sensitisation among humans[27]: a maximisation test of 4% fennel oil in petrolatum produced no sensitisation reaction in 24 volunteers.
Phototoxicity[27]: no phototoxicity reactions reported on hairless mice and swine.
Subchronic toxicity[23]: total protein significantly reduced in testes and vas deferens and increased in the seminal vesicles and prostate gland. Alkaline phosphatase was also decreased in male rats receiving 100 mg/day oral fennel seed extract for 15 days. The same dose

administered to females for 10 days lead to vaginal cornification and oestrous. The mean weights of the oviduct, endometrium, myometrium, cervix and vagina were also increased. The findings were attributed to oestrogenic-like activity of the extract.

100 mg/kg/day fennel fruit extract in drinking water for 90 days caused significant body weight gain in male mice and weight loss in females. Alopecia was observed in 3/10 males, swollen testes in 1/10 males and penile erection in 2/10. No toxic symptoms observed in females. No adverse effects on reproductive system reported.

Mutagenicity: fennel oil and trans-anethole are mutagenic in Ames strains TA 98 and TA 100 in presence of activation system. (Few details provided).[24]

Water or methanol extract negative in Ames strains TA 89 and TA 100 and in Bacillus subtilis rec assay. (Few details provided)[25]

(Bitter fennel oil)[28]

LD50 oral in rats: 4.52 ml/Kg*

LD50 dermal in rabbits: 5 ml/Kg*

Primary skin irritation: Undiluted is not irritating to hairless mice*.

Applied for 24-hours under occlusion to intact or abraded rabbit skin: irritating.*

Diluted 4% in petrolatum produced no irritation after a 48-hour closed patch tests on human volunteers.*

Sensitisation among humans[28]: a maximisation test of 4% bitter fennel oil in petrolatum produced 3 sensitisation reactions in 25 volunteers.*

A maximisation test of 4% bitter fennel oil in petrolatum produced no sensitisation reactions in 29 volunteers[29].

* Test performed with deteriorated (oxidised) oil

(Estragole)

Estragole is carcinogenic in mice, inducing hepatomas, and is mutagenic in some system and forms DNA adducts *in vivo* and *in vitro*[31]

Databases used

CA Search 1967-96, Medline 1966-96, Embase 1974-96, Ref. Tox. Eff. Chem. Sub., Toxline, Biosis, HDSB.

Keywords

Foeniculum vulgare

Evaluation and remarks

Cat. C (Fennel)

Cat. C (Bitter fennel)

General references

1. Index Kewensis, Clarendon Press

2. Penso G., Index Plantarum Medicinalium Totius Mundi Eorumque Synonymorum, OEMF, 1983

3. European Commission Decision 96/335/EC of 8 May 1996, Official Journal of the European Community No. L132 of 1 June 1996

4. International Cosmetic Ingredient Dictionary 6th ed., CTFA, *1*, 1995

5. Benigni R., Capra C., Cattorini P.E., Piante Medicinali chimica farmacologia e terapia, Inverni & Della Beffa, *1*, 605-607, 1971
6. Comprehensive Licensing Standards of Cosmetics by Category, Yakuji Nippo Ltd., 2, 206, 1987
7. Council of Europe, Flavouring substances and natural sources of flavourings 3rd ed. Maisonneuve, (200, 201, N2), 1981
8. Fenaroli G., Sostanze Aromatiche Naturali, Hoepli ed., 562-567, 1963
9. Flavouring Extract Manufactures Association (Fema), Survey of flavouring ingredients usage levels, (No. 2481, 2482, 2483) Food Technology, 173 (275), 1965
10. Grieve M., A modern herbal, Barnes & Noble Books, *1*, 293-298, 1996
11. Guenther E., the essential oils, D. Van Nostrand, *4*, 634-645, 1952
12. The Japanese Cosmetic Ingredients Codex, Yakuji Nippo, LTD. 295, 1993
13. Leung A.Y., Foster S., Encyclopedia of common natural ingredients, Wiley & Son Publ., 240-243, 1996
14. Martindale 31st ed., The Royal Pharmaceutical Society, 1996
15. Merck Index 12th ed., Merck & Co. Inc., 1996
16. Monographs Foeniculi aetheroleum and Foeniculi fructus, Bundesanzeiger, No. 74 (Apr.19,1991) and No. 94 (Apr. 19, 1991), through Le monografie tedesche, Studio Edizioni, *1*, 1991
17. Monograph Foeniculi fructus, European Scientific Cooperative for Phyto therapy (ESCOP), 1996
18. Paris R.R., Moyse H., Matière Médicale 2nd ed., Masson, *2*, 474-475,1981
19. Proserpio G., Martelli A., Patri G.F., Elementi di fitocosmesi, Sepem, *2*, 686-687, 1982
20. Van Hellemont J., Compendium de Phytotherapie, APB, 162-164, 1986
21. Wichtl M., Teedrogen, WVG, 171-173, 1989

Specific references

22. Albert- Puleo M., Fennel and Anise as Estrogenic Agent, J. of Ethnopharmacol., *2*, 337-344, 1980
23. Malini et al., Ind. J. Physiol. Pharmacol., *29*, 21-26, 1985, through Chem. Abs. 103: 17227a, 1985
24. Marcus C., Lichtenstein. E. P., J. Agric. Food Chem., *30*, 563-568, 1982
25. Morimoto et al., Mutation Research., *97*, 81-102, 1982
26. Nater J.P., De Groot A.C., Unwanted Effects of cosmetic and drugs used in Dermatology, Excerpta Medica, 314- 318, 1983
27. Opdyke. D.L.J., Food and Cosmetics Toxicology, *12*, 879, 1974
28. Opdyke. D.L.J., Food and Cosmetics Toxicology, *14*, 4S, 309, 1976
29. Opdyke. D.L.J., Food and Cosmetics Toxicology, *17*, 5, 529, 1978

30. Shah et al., J. of Ethnopharmacol., *34*, 167-172, 1991
31. Recommendations concerning undesirable active principles, 3.7, 28th meeting Committee of Experts on Cosmetic Products, Rome, 3-7 November 1997, Council of Europe.
32. DAB 10
33. OAB '90
34. Ph. Helv. VII
35. FU IX
36. Ph. B. V
37. Ph. Ned. 8
38. Ph. F. X

Gentiana lutea

Botanical name[1]	*Gentiana lutea* L.
Botanical synonyms[2]	*Asterias lutea* Bork.
Botanical family	Gentianaceae
Common names	Bitterwort (English) Gele Gentiaan (Dutch) Kultakatkero (Finnish) Gentiane jaune (French) Gelber Enzian (German) Genziana (Italian) Gulsoterot (Norwegian) Genciana (Spanish) Gullgentiana (Swedish)
EU INCI name[3]	*Gentiana lutea*
CTFA INCI name[4]	Gentian (*Gentiana lutea*) Gentian (*Gentiana lutea*) extract

CAS number	72968-42-4
EINECS number	277-139-0
Parts used	Rhyzomes and roots

Important constituents including active principles[12, 16, 17]
- Essential oil (traces)[17]
- Bitter glycosides (1.1-3.5%)[17] (secoiridoids: gentiopicrin, swertia-marin, amarogentin (0.05%)[17], amaroswerin)
- Polyphenols (xanthone glycosides: gentisin and isogentisin, gentiosin, 1,3,7-trimethoxyxanthone)
- Polysaccharides (pectins)
- Oligosaccharides (saccharose, gentiobiose (5-8%)[18], gentianose)
- Monosaccharides (fructose, glucose, mannose)
- Triterpenes (β-amyrine, lupeol)
- Amino acids (alanine, asparagine, glutamine)
- Alkaloids (gentianine (0.6-0.8%)[16], gentialutine)

Preparation
1) Glycolic extract E/D = 5:1
2) Tincture T/D = 5:1
3) Dry extract E/D = 1:5

Manufacturing process
1) Percolation with propylene glycol 50%
2) Maceration with alcohol 60%
3) Percolation with water and concentration under vacuum to dryness

Examples of specifications[19]   1) pH: 4.5 to 6.0
Relative density at 20°: 1.038 to 1.044
Refractive index at 20°: 1.385 to 1.395
Dry residue: 0.5 to 1.5%
Heavy metals ≤ 5 ppm
2) Dry residue: not less than 5%
3) Loss on drying: less than 4%

Intended cosmetic effects and used concentration in cosmetic products
Tonic, soothing, purifying

(Glycolic extract)
Up to 7% in products for sensitive, impure, oily skin and scalp Other possible effects Traditionally used on insect bites, bruises, wounds, as lenitive and granulation promoting agent

Main toxicological data[21]   Mutagenicity. An aqueous extract (5mg/plate) caused a 7 and 4 fold increase in revertants in Salmonella strains TA 100 in the presence and absence of metabolic activation respectively.
A methanol extract (10 mg/plate) caused a threefold increase in revertants in strain TA 100.
Both types of extract were negative in Salmonella strain TA 98. The aqueous but not the methanol extract was judged weakly positive in Bacillus subtilis rec-assay in the absence of metabolic activation DNA repair Bacillus subtilis: 100 g/l (RTECS)

Databases used   CA Search 1967-95, Medline 1966-96, Embase 1974-95, Ref. Tox. Eff. Chem. Sub., Toxline, Biosis, HDSB,

Keywords   *Gentiana lutea*

Evaluation and remarks   **Cat. B**

General references   1. Index Kewensis, Clarendon Press
2. Penso G., Index Plantarum Medicinalium Totius Mundi Eorumque Synonymorum, OEMF, 1983
3. European Commission Decision 96/335/CE of 8 May 1996, Official Journal of the European Community No. L132 of 1 June 1996
4. International Cosmetic Ingredient Dictionary 6th ed., CTFA, *1*, 1995
5. Benigni R., Capra C., Cattorini P.E., Piante Medicinali chimica farmacologia e terapia, Inverni & Della Beffa, *1*, 646-653, 1971
6. Comprehensive Licensing Standards of Cosmetics by Category, Yakuji Nippo Ltd., *2*, 208, 1987
7. Council of Europe, Flavouring substances and natural sources of flavourings 3rd ed. Maisonneuve, (214, N 2), 1981
8. Fenaroli G., Sostanze Aromatiche Naturali, Hoepli ed., 244, 1963
9. Flavouring Extract Manufactures Association (Fema), Survey of flavouring ingredients usage levels, (No. 2506) Food Technology, 174 , *2*, 1965

10. Grieve M., A modern herbal, Barnes & Noble Books, 347-349, 1996
11. Japanese Cosmetic Ingredients Dictionary, 3
12. Leung A.Y., Foster S., Encyclopedia of common natural ingredients, Wiley & Son Publ., 267-269, 1995
13. Martindale 31st ed., The Royal Pharmaceutical Society, 1996
14. Merck Index 12th ed., Merck & Co. Inc., 1996
15. Monographs Gentianae radix, Bundesanzeiger, No. 223 (Nov. 30, 1985) and No. 50 (Mar 10, 1990), through Le monografie tedesche, Studio Edizioni, 4, 1996
16. Newall C., Anderson L., Phillipson J.D., Herbal Medicines: a guide for health care professionals, The Pharmaceutical Press, 134, 1996
17. Van Hellemont J., Compendium de Phytotherapie, APB, 176-177, 1986
18. Wichtl M., Teedrogen, WVG, 153-155, 1989

Specific references

19. Indena Product Specification, 1996
20. Heath H.B., Herbs – Their use in cosmetics and toiletries, Cosm. and Toilet., 92, 19-24, 1977
21. Morimoto I. et al., Mutation Research, 97, 81-102, 1982
22. Nater J.P., De Groot A.C., Unwanted Effects of cosmetic and drugs used in Dermatology, Excerpta Medica, 319, 1983
23. BP '88
24. BPC '73
25. BHP '90
26. OAB
27. Ph. B. V
28. Ph. Eu. III
29. Ph. Fr. IX
30. FU IX
31. DAB 9
32. Ph. Helv. VII

Glycine soja

Botanical name[1]	*Glycine max* (L.) Merr.
Botanical synonyms[2]	*Glycine soja* Sieb et Zucc., *G. hispida* Maxim., *Dolichos soja* L., *Phaseolus max* L., *Soja angustifolia* Miq., *Soja hispida* Moench., *Soja max* Piper
Botanical family	Leguminosae
Common names	Soybean (English) Sojaboon (Dutch) Soija (Finnish) Soya (French) Sojabohne (German) Soia (Italian) Soja (Spanish) Soja (Swedish)
EU INCI name[3]	*Glycine soja*
CTFA INCI name[4]	Soybean (*Glycine soja*) extract Soybean (*Glycine soja*) germ extract Soybean (*Glycine soja*) unsaponifiables Soybean (*Glycine soja*) protein Soybean (*Glycine soja*) sterol Lecithin
CAS number	84776-91-0 (germ extract) 91770-67-1 (unsaponifiables) 9010-10-0 (protein) 8002-43-5 (lecithin)
EINECS number	294-853-8 (unsaponifiables) 232-720-8 (protein) 232-307-2 (lecithin)
Parts used	Seeds

Important constituents including active principles[10, 11]

- Triglycerides (about 20%)[11] (containing linoleic, oleic, linolenic, palmitic and stearic acids)
- Proteins (about 40%)[10] albumins (mainly legumelin and soy legumelin), globulins (mainly glycinin and phaseolin) and casein
- Amino acids (triptophan, lysine, methionine, cysteine)
- Phospholipids:
  Lecithin (up to 5%) containing: (phosphatidylcholine (about 70%), phosphatidylethanolamine (up to 7%), phosphatidylinosi-

tol, phosphatidic acid) and (palmitic 11.7%, stearic 4%, palmitoleic 8.6%, oleic 9.8%, linoleic 55%, linolenic 4%, C_{20} to C_{22} 5.5% acids)[10.]

Cephalins

- Triterpene saponins
- Unsaponifiables[15.] (about 1-1.5%) (campesterol 25%, stigmasterol 25%, sistosterol 50%)
- Anthocyanes
- Isoflavonglycosides (genistin, daidzin, methylgenistin)
- Sugars (15-25%)[11.] (saccharose, raffinose, pentosans and galactosans)
- Polysaccharides (stachyose)
- Starch
- Carotenoids
- Vitamins (0.2-0.5%) (mainly B_1, B_2, PP, E, C)
- Mineral salts

Preparation

1)[5, 7.] Soy extract
2) Unsaponifiables
3)[8.] Soybean phospolipid

Manufacturing process

1)[5.] Liquid prepared by adding purified water to a powder from the seeds obtained through boiling, grinding and then filtering
2) Saponification and partition betwen butylalcohol and exane
3)[10.] By-product of the manufacturing of soybean oil

Examples of specifications

1)[5.] pH: 6.0-7.0
Heavy metals: not more than 20 ppm.
Arsenic: not more than 2 ppm
Residue on ignition: 1.5-4.0%
2)[15.] Saponification number: < 25
Iodine number: 135-160
Acid number: < 6
Peroxide number: < 40
Tocopherols: 10%
Sterols: 40-65%
Carotenoids: 0.025%
3)[8.] Acid value: not more than 40%
Benzene-insoluble substances: not more than 0.3%
Acetone-soluble substances: not more than 40%
Heavy metals: not more than 20 ppm.
Arsenic: not more than 2 ppm
Loss on drying: not more than 2%

Intended cosmetic effects and used concentration in cosmetic products

(extract)
Up to 0.5%
Skin protectant, moisturising, soothing, smoothing

(protein)
Hair conditioning agent, emollient, smoothing, skin protectant

(unsaponifiables)
Up to 2%
Emollient, emulsifier, soothing, moisturising

(lecithin)
Up to 5%
Moisturising, hair-conditioning agent, emulsifier

Other possible effects

Antioxidant

(unsaponifiables)
Stimulation of collagen and increase of skin elasticity, wound healing

Main toxicological data

(soytoxin)[13]
LD $_{50}$ i.p in mice: 7-8 mg/kg b.w.
Soybean seed containsthe toxic agglutinin PHASIN, which is denatured by cooking[17]

(unsaponifiables)[15]
LD $_0$ oral in mice: > 10000 mg/kg
LD $_{50}$ i.p in mice: 4000 mg/kg

Databases used

CA Search 1967-95, Medline 1966-95, Embase 1974-95, Ref. Tox. Eff. Chem. Sub., Toxline, Toxbio, Toxcas

Keywords

Glycine max or *Glycine soja,* extract or unsaponifiables, cosmetic

Evaluation and remarks

Cat. A (extract; insaponifiables; phospholids)

Some soybean extracts might contain isoflavons and phyto-oestrogens, the oral use of which is currently under research among menopausal women. In the case of external use, there are no toxic elements and penetration of isoflavons should be virtually nil.

General references

1. Index Kewensis, Clarendon Press
2. Penso G., Index Plantarum Medicinalium Totius Mundi Eorumque Synonymorum, OEMF, 1983
3. European Commission Decision 96/335/EC of 8 May 1996, Official Journal of the European Community No. L132 of 1 June 1996
4. International Cosmetic Ingredient Dictionary 6th ed., CTFA, 1995
5. Comprehensive Licensing Standards of Cosmetics by Category, Yakuji Nippo Ltd., *4*, 357, 1989
6. Council of Europe, Flavouring substances and natural sources of flavourings 3rd ed. Maisonneuve, (217 N2), 1981
7. The Japanese Cosmetic Ingredients Codex, ed. Yakuji Nippo Ltd., 839, 1993
8. The Japanese Standards of Cosmetic Ingredients 2nd ed., Yakuji Nippo Ltd., 1985
9. Martindale 31st ed., The Royal Pharmaceutical Society, 1996
10. Merck Index 12th ed., Merck & Co. Inc., 1996

11. Paris R.R., Moyse H., Matière Médicale, Masson 2nd ed., *2*, 393-394 and 398-401, 1981

12. Proserpio G., Martelli A., Patri G.F., Elementi di fitocosmesi, Sepem, *2*, 787-788; 819, 1983

Specific references

13. Datasheet of German delegation 10/96

14. Eggensperger, Pflanzliche Wirkstoffe für Kosmetika, Melcher Verlag GmbH, 1995

15. Expanscience-Chimie Technical documentations

16. Gessner, Gift+ Arzneipflanzer, 3 ed, 1974

17. Hänsel R. et al (eds.), Hagers Handbuch der pharmazeutischen Praxis, 5th ed. 1993

18. Hoppe, Drogenkunde, 8th ed, 1975

19. Schneider M., Lecithin- Einsatz und Wirkungsweise in Kosmetischen Zubereitungen, Seifen-Öle-Fette-Wachse, *111*, 1,16,1985

20. Zander, Pflanzennamen, 15 ed, 1974

21. BP 88

22. USP XXII

Lilium candidum

Botanical name[1]	*Lilium candidum* L.
Botanical synonyms	-
Botanical family	Liliaceae
Common names	White lily (English)
	Witte Lelie (Dutch)
	Madonnalilja (Finnish)
	Lis blanc (French)
	Weisse Lilie (German)
	Giglio bianco (Italian)
	Madonnalilje (Norwegian)
	Lirio común (Spanish)
EU INCI name[2]	*Lilium candidum*
CTFA INCI name[3]	White lily (*Lilium candidum*) extract

CAS number	84776-67-0
EINECS number	283-996-1
Parts used	Bulbs and flowers

Important constituents including active principles[5]

- Essential oil (0.3%)[5]:
  (Vanilline (up to 2.5)[5]
  π-hydroxy-m-methoxytoluene (till 50%)[5]
  π-cresol, linalol, terpineol, phenylethylalcohol and their ester with acetic, palmitic, benzoic, propionic and cinnamic acids)
- Amino acids (γ-methyleneglutamic, γ-methylglutamic acids and γ-methylenebutyrolactone)
- Flavonoids (kaempferol, kaempferol glycosides, luteolin-7-glucoside)[19]
- Flavone alkaloid (lilaline)
- Pyrroline alkaloids (jatropham, ethyljatropham, citraconimide)[17, 13]
- Phytosterols
- Organic acids (citric, malic, succinic, oxalic and piruvic acids)
- Phenol acids (chlorogenic acid)
- Starch (about 14% in bulbs)14.
- Polysaccharides (glucomannan)
- Carotenoids (b-carotene, cryptoxanthin, echinenone-like carotenoid, zeaxanthin, capsanthin, capsorubin)
- Tannins
- Mineral salts

– Vitamins (mainly C)

Preparation
1) Glycolic extract from bulbs[4.]
2) Hydroglycolic extract from flowers[16.]

Manufacturing process
1) Extraction of bulbs with purified water, ethanol, propylene glycol, 1,3-butylene glycol or mixture of these[4.]
2) Extraction of flowers with propylene glycol 50% and concentration under vacuum to final E/D ratio 10:1[16.].

Examples of specifications
1)[4.] Heavy metals: not more than 20 ppm
Arsenic: not more than 2 ppm
2)[16.] pH: 6.0 to 6.5
Relative density at 20°C: 1.035 to 1.042
Refractive index at 20°C: 1.386 to 1.390
Dry residue: 0.1 to 0.8%

Intended cosmetic effects and used concentration in cosmetic products
Soothing, emollient, moisturising, protective
Up to 10% in detergents, gels, solutions, emulsions, masks for ageing, dry and chapped skin, in pre- and after-sun products

Other possible effects
Anti-irritant, free radical scavenger, microvessel protectant, antimicotic. Anti-UV erythema. Also used on wounds and burns, insect bites, swollen skin, dislocations (traditional use of olive oil extract)[11.]

Main toxicological data[10.]
Primary skin irritation in rabbits: non-irritant
Acute eye irritation in rabbits: non-irritant

Databases used
CA Search 1967-95, Medline 1966-95, Embase 1974-95, Ref. Tox. Eff. Chem. Sub., Toxline, IPA, Embase, Biosis, Scisearch

Keywords
Lilium candidum, Lily

Evaluation and remarks
Cat. B

General references
1. Index Kewensis, Clarendon Press
2. European Commission Decision 96/335/EC of 8 May 1996, Official Journal of the European Community No. L132 of 1 June 1996
3. International Cosmetic Ingredient Dictionary 6th *ed.*, 2,CTFA, 1995
4. Cosmetic Licensing Standards of Cosmetics by Category, Yakuji Nippo Ltd., 1, 154, 1986
5. Fenaroli G., Le sostanze aromatiche, Hoepli ed., 603-604, 1963
6. Grieve M., A modern herbal, Barnes & Noble Books, *2*, 482-484, 1996
7. The Japanese Cosmetic Ingredients Codex, Yakuji Nippo Ltd., 444, 1993
8. Proserpio G., Martelli A., Patri G.F., Elementi di fitocosmesi, Sepem, *2*, 497, 1983

Specific references
9. Avalle N., L'estratto di bulbo di giglio ed il suo impiego in cosmetologia, Rivista Italiana EPPOS, *54*, 1, 1972

10. Indena's reports
11. German delegation data sheets, October, 1996
12. Eisenreichovà E., Haladovà M., Buckovà A., Ubik K., Uhrìn D., Derivatives of pyrroline in Lilium candidum L., Chem. Papers *45*, 5, 709-711, 1991
13. Eisenreichovà E., Haladovà M., Buckovà A., Tomko J., Uhrìn D., Ubik K., A pyrroline-pyrrolidine alkaloid from Lilium candidum bulbs, Phytochemistry *31*, 3, 1084-1085, 1992
14. Hansel R. et al., Hagers Handbuch der pharmazeutischen Praxis, 5, 1993
15. Hoppe, Drogenkunde, *8*, 1975
16. Indena Product Specifications
17. Nater J.P., De Groot A.C., Unwanted effects of cosmetic and drugs used in dermatology, Excerpta Medica, 315, 1983
18. Zander, Pflanzennamen 15, 1994
19. Nagi É., Neszmélyi A, Verzár-Petri G., Characteristic flavonoids of Lilium candidum L. and their distribution in different plant parts, Flavonoids and Bioflavonoids, 1985.

Medicago sativa

Botanical name[1]	*Medicago sativa* L.
Botanical synonyms[1]	*Medicago falcata* L.
Botanical family	Fabaceae
Common names	Alfalfa (English)
	Lucerne (Dutch)
	Sinimailanen (Finnish)
	Luzerne (French)
	Luzerne (German)
	Erba medica (Italian)
	Blålusern (Norwegian)
	Trébol (Spanish)
	Blålusern (Swedish)
EU INCI name[2]	*Medicago sativa*
CTFA INCI name[3]	Alfalfa (*Medicago sativa*) extract

CAS number	84082-36-0
EINECS number	281-984-0
Parts used	Aerial parts

Important constituents including active principles[7, 8, 11]

- Triterpene saponins (up to 3%)[7] (medicagosides A, C, G, I, J) and aglycones (medicagenic acid, soyasapogenols A, B, C, D, E, F and hederagenin)
- Isoflavonoids (tricin, biochanin A, daidzein, formononetin, genistein, coumestrol)
- Isoflavans (sativan, 5'-methoxysativan)
- Coumarins (medicagol, coumestrol, sativol, trifoliol, lucernol, daphnoretin)
- Tannins
- Phytosterols (α- and β-sitosterol, campesterol, cycloartenol, α- and β-spinasterol, stigmasterol) and their esters with palmitic, lauric and myristic acids
- Triglycerides (cont. linoleic, linolenic and palmitic acids)
- Sugars (arabinose, fructose, sucrose, xylose, rhamnose, glucose, galactose)
- Glucuronic acid
- Pectins
- Starch
- Vitamins (B1, B2, B6, B12, C, E, H, K, PP)

- Amino acids (asparagine, arginine, cystine, histidine, isoleucine, leucine, lysine, methionine, phenylalanine, threonine, thryptophan, valine, inosine, adenine, adenosine)
- Proteins 15%[7]
- Non-protein aminoacid (canavanine) up to 1.5% of the dry weight
- Alcohols (octacosanol, triaconatol)
- Polyalcohol (inositol)
- Organic acids (maleic, malic, malonic, oxalic, citric, quinic)
- Hydrocarbons (nonacosane, triacontane, hentriacontane)
- Pigments (chlorophyll, xanthophylls, β-carotene, anthocyanins, cryptoxanthin, violaxanthin, zeaxanthin, neoxanthin)
- Inosine
- Mineral salts 1-2%[11] (calcium, aluminum, cobalt, iron, magnesium, manganese, phosphorus, copper, zinc, potassium)
- Alkaloids (stachydrine, homostachydrine) (trigonelline only in seeds)

Preparation

1) Fluid extract E/D = 1:1[8]
2) Dry extract E/D = 1:4[11]

Manufacturing process

1) Percolation with alcohol 25% and concentration under vacuum to final E/D ratio 1:1
2) Percolation with alcohol 25% and concentration under vacuum to dryness

Examples of specifications   -

Intended cosmetic effects and used concentration in cosmetic products

Tonic, anti-ageing, firming, protective, moisturising; flavour, fragrance
In products for ageing skin and in facial masks

Other possible effects

Antimicrobial, granulation-promoting agent (unsaponifiable fraction), estrogenic, hemolytic

Main toxicological data[9]

(canavanine) [RTECS]
LD_0 in rats: 10 mg/kg
Induces a systemic lupus erythematosus-like syndrome in female monkeys.[9]

(saponins)[9]
Dietary studies in rats and monkeys showed no evidence of toxicity. Serum lipid levels were lowered.
Mutagenicity (*Salmonella* strains TA98 and TA 100): negative.

Databases used

CA Search 1967-96, Medline 1966-96, Embase 1974-96, Reg. Tox. Eff. Chem. Sub.

Keywords

Medicago sativa, Alfalfa, Lucerne

Evaluation and remarks   **Cat. B**

General references

1. Index Kewensis, Clarendon Press

2. European Commission Decision 96/335/EC of 8 May 1996, Official Journal of the European Community No. L132 of 1 June 1996
3. International Cosmetic Ingredient Dictionary 6th ed., CTFA, *1*, 1995
4. Council of Europe, Flavouring substances and natural sources of flavourings (274, N2), 3rd ed., Maisonneuve, 1981
5. Flavouring Extract Manufacturers Association (Fema), GRAS Substances, reprinted from Food Technology, (257) 155, February 1965
6. Grieve M., A modern herbal, Barnes & Noble Books, 2 501, 1996
7. Leung A.Y., Foster S., Encyclopedia of common natural ingredients, Wiley & Son Publ., 15-17, 1996
8. Martindale 31st ed., The Royal Pharmaceutical Society, 1996
9. Newall C.A., Anderson L.A., Phillipson J.D., Herbal Medicines, The Pharmaceutical Press, 23-24, 1996
10. Paris R.R., Moyse H., Matière Médicale 2nd ed., Masson, *2*, 391,1981
11. Van Hellemont J., Compendium de Phytotherapie, APB, 248-249,1986

Specific references

12. Beckstrom-Sternberg S.M., Duke J.A., "The Phytochemical Database"
13. Datasheet: Medicago sativa RD 5/7-27
14. De Froment, Unsaponifiable substance from alfalfa for pharmaceutical and cosmetic use, Fr. Demande 2,187,328, 22nd Feb 1974
15. De Navarre MG, The chemistry and manufacture of cosmetics, 2nd ed., Allured Pub. Cie., 1975
16. Hudson B.J.F., Mahgoub S.E.O., Naturally-occurring antioxidants in Leaf Lipids, J. Sci. Food Agric., *31*, 646-650, 1980
17. Malinow M.R. et al., the Toxicity of Alfalfa Saponins in rats, Food Cosmet. Toxicol., *19*, 443-445, 1981
18. BHP 1983

Melaleuca alternifolia

Botanical name[1]	*Melaleuca alternifolia* Cheel
Botanical synonyms	*Melaleuca linariifolia* var. *alternifolia* Sm.
Botanical family	Myrtaceae
Common name	Tea tree (English)
	Teepuu (Finnish)
	Melaleuca alternifolia (French)
	Tétre (Norwegian)
	Arbol del té (Spanish)
	Tea tree (Swedish)
EU INCI name[2]	*Melaleuca alternifolia*
CTFA INCI name[3]	Tea tree (*Melaleuca alternifolia*) oil

CAS number	85085-48-9
	8022-72-8 (essential oil)
	68647-73-4 (essential oil)
EINECS number	285-377-1
Parts used	Fresh leaves and branches

Important constituents including active principles[5]
– Essential oil (1-2%):
(Monoterpenes: α-pinene, α-thujene, β-pinene, π-cymene, sabinene, myrcene, α- and β-phellandrene, α-terpinene, limonene, cineole (less than 15%)[7], γ-terpinene, π-cymene, terpinolene, linalool, α-terpineol, terpinen-4-ol (more than 30%)[7], globulol
Sesquiterpenes: aromadendrene, viridiflorene, d-cadinene and sesquiterpene alcohols

Preparation Essential oil (Tea tree oil)

Manufacturing process Steam distillation of leaves and branches

Examples of specifications[5, 11] Specific gravity at 15°C: 0.8950 to 0.9050
Specific optical rotation: +6°48' to +9°48' Refractive index at 20°: 1.4760 to 1.4810 Ester number: 2 to 7 Ester number after acetylation: 80 to 90
Terpinen-n-ol: not less than 30% Cineole content: less than 10% Solubility in 80% alcohol (w/w): soluble in 0.6 to 0.8 vol.

Intended cosmetic effects and used concentration in cosmetic products

Tonic, deodorant, purifying, flavour, fragrance

Up to 0.5% in toothpastes and mouthwashes for gums and mucosae

Up to 2% in creams for chapped and impure skin, hands and nails, deodorants

Up to 3% in bath preparations, shampoos and special detergents.

Other possible effects[10]

Antiseptic (against bacteria and fungi), stimulant, hyperemic, anti-acnes, analgesic, creams and lotions for relief of sore muscles, preservative (secondary)

Main toxicological data[11, 12]

LD_{50} oral in rats: > 1 900mg/kg

LD_{50} dermal on rabbits: > 5 000 mg/kg

Primary skin irritation on rabbits (Draize method) on abraded and intact skin:the index was 5 (severe irritant).

As part of an acute dermal LD_{50} study, the undiluted material produced irritant effects and skin abnormalities at necropsy in rabbits patch-tested for 24 hours under occlusion at a dose of 5 000 mg/kg.

30-day skin irritation in rabbits (25% concentration in liquid paraffin): slight initial irritation, reducing to 0 by week 2.

21-day skin cumulative irritancy patch test in humans: 5 out of 28 subjects exhibited slight erythema. Contact allergy has been reported in 2 patients. Systemic contact dermatitis has been reported in 1 patient.

A 48-hour closed-patch test at a concentration of 1% in petrolatum on the backs of 22 volunteers produced no irritation.

Sensitisation in guinea pigs: not sensitising.

A maximisation test on human (22 volunteers): the material was tested at a concentration of 1% in petrolatum and produced no sensitisation reactions.

Mutagenicity (Ames test): not mutagenic.

Phototoxicity. At a concentration of 100%, it did not produce phototoxic effects when applied to the skin of hairless mice but some irritation was noted.

Allergenicity data are reported.[13, 14]

(Eucalyptol or 1,8-cineole or p-cineole)

has been studied sub-chronically in rats and mice; a NOEL of 300 mg/kg bw has been established. Eucalyptol has been found non mutagenic in different systems[15]

Databases

CA Search 1967-95, Medline 1966-95, Embase 1974-95, Ref. Tox. Eff. Cosm. Sub., Biosis, Excerpta Medica, Biological Abstract, Pascal, FSTA, Toxline

Keywords

Melaleuca alternifolia, Tea tree oil

Evaluation and remarks

Cat. A

General references

1. Index Kewensis, Clarendon Press
2. European Commission Decision 96/335/EC of 8 May 1996, Official Journal of the European Community No. L132 of 1 June 1996
3. International Cosmetic Ingredient Dictionary 6th ed., CTFA, *2*, 1995
4. Council of Europe, Flavouring substances and natural sources of flavourings 3rd ed. Maisonneuve, (275, N3), 1981
5. Guenther E., The Essential oil, D. Van Nostrand, *4*, 526-541, 1958
6. Martindale 31st ed., The Royal Pharmaceutical Society, 1996
7. Leung A.Y., Foster S., Encyclopedia of common natural ingredients, Wiley & Son Publ., 110-111, 1996

Specific references

8. Altman P.M., Australian tea tree oil, Austr. J. Pharmacy, *69*, 276-278, 1988
9. Brophy J.J., Davies N.W., Southwell I. A., Stiff I.A., Williams L.R., Gas Chromatographic quality control for oil of Melaleuca Terpinen-4-ol type (Australian tea tree), J. Agric. Food Chem., *37*, 1330-1335, 1989
10. Carson C.F., Riley T.V., Antimicrobial activity of the essential oil of Melaleuca alternifolia, Letters Appl. Microbiol., *16*, 49-55, 1993
11. Main Camp specifications
12. Opdyke D.L.J., Food and Chemical Toxicology, 26, 407, 1988
13. Selvaag E., Eriksen B.,thune P., Contact allergy due tea tree oil and cross-sensitisation to colophony, Contact Dermatitis, *31*, 124,1994
14. Knight T.E., Hausen B.M., Melaleuca oil (tea tree oil) dermatitis, Journ. Amer. Acad. Derm., *30*, 3, 423-427, 1994
15. Recommendations concerning undesirable active principles, 3.8, 28th meeting Committee of Experts on Cosmetic Products, Rome, 3-7 November 1997, Council of Europe.
16. BPC '49

Melaleuca leucadendron

Botanical name[1]	*Melaleuca leucadendron* L. var. *minor* Sm.
Botanical synonyms[2]	*Melaleuca minor* Sm.
Botanical family	Myrtaceae
Common name	Cajeput tree (English)
	Cajeputboom (Dutch)
	Kajeputpuu (Finnish)
	Cajeputier (French)
	Kajeputbaum (German)
	Cajeput (Italian)
	Kajeput (Norwegian)
	Cayeput (Spanish)
	Kajeput (Swedish)
EU INCI name	-
CTFA INCI name	-

CAS number	85480-37-1
	8008-98-8 (essential oil)
EINECS/ELINCS number	287-316-4
Parts used	Fresh leaves, branches and twigs

Important constituents including active principles[7, 8, 18.]

– Essential oil (up to 1%):
(Monoterpenes: α- and β-pinene, β-thujene, limonene, π-cymene, α-terpinene, δ-elemene, β-elemene, aromadendrene, α-humulene, cadinene, dipentene, linalool, geraniol, terpinen-4-ol (up to 47%)8., α-terpineol and esters, cineole (14-65%)8.
Sesquiterpenes: α-bisabolene, β-cariophyllene, azulene
Sesquiterpene alcohols
Aldehydes: valeraldehyde, benzaldehyde
Organic acids: butyric, valeric, benzoic acids)
Phenol derivative: 3,5-dimethyl-4,6-di-0-methylphloroacetophenone

Preparation[7.]	Essential oil (Cajeput oil, syn. Cajuput oil)
Manufacturing process[7.]	Steam distillation of the fresh leaves and branches
Examples of specifications[7.]	Specific gravity at 15°C: 0.917 to 0.930
	Specific optical rotation: up to -3°40'
	Refractive index at 20°C: 1.466 to 1.472

Cineole content: 50-60%

Solubility: soluble in 1 vol. of 80% alcohol. Occasionally soluble in 2.5 to 3 vol. of 70% alcohol

Intended cosmetic effects and used concentration In cosmetic products[18]

Tonic, deodorant, purifying; fragrance

Up to 0.1% in soaps, detergents, creams and lotions, deodorants, sports massage oils and liniments, creams and lotion for impure, atonic skin.

Other possible effects[18]

Stimulant, hyperemic, antiseptic; external remedy for rheumatism, insecticide, analgesic in toothache

Main toxicological data[17]

LD_{50} oral in rats: 3 870 mg/kg

LD_{50} dermal in rabbits: > 5 000mg/kg

Primary skin irritation on hairless mice, 24 hours under occlusion swine and rabbits (undiluted essential oil): non-irritant.

Patch test on humans: non irritant when tested 4% in petrolatum for 48-hours.

Sensitisation in humans: not sensitising when tested at 4% in petrolatum.

Phototoxicity (on hairless mice and swine): no phototoxic effects have been reported.

(Eucalyptol or 1,8-cineole or p-cineole)

has been studied sub-chronically in rats and mice; a NOEL of 300 mg/kg bw has been established. Eucalyptol has been found non mutagenic in different systems.[19]

Databases used

CA Search 1967-95, Medline 1966-95, Embase 1974-95, Ref. Tox. Eff. Chem. Sub., Toxline, Excerpta Medica, Biological Abstracts

Keywords

Melaleuca leucadendra, Cajeput oil

Evaluation and remarks

Cat: A

General references

1. Index Kewensis, Clarendon Press
2. Penso G., Index Plantarum Medicinalium Totius Mundi Eorumque Synonymorum, OEMF, 1983
3. Council of Europe, Flavouring substances and natural sources of flavourings, 3rd ed. Maisonneuve (276, N2), 1981
4. Fenaroli G., Sostanze Aromatiche Naturali, Hoepli ed., 422-423, 1963
5. Flavouring Extract Manufacturers Association (Fema), Survey of flavouring ingredients usage levels, (No. 2225), Food Technology, 2, (265), 1965
6. Grieve M., A modern herbal, Barnes & Noble Books, *1*, 151, 1996
7. Guenther E., The Essential oils, D. Van Nostrand, *4*, 542-548, 1958
8. Leung A.Y., Foster S., Encyclopedia of common natural ingredients, Wiley & Son Publ., 110-111, 1996
9. Martindale 31st ed., The Royal Pharmaceutical Society, 1996

10. Merck Index 12th ed., Merck & Co. Inc., 1996
11. Paris R.R., Moyse H., Matière Médicale, Masson ed., *2*, 447, 1981
12. Van Hellemont J., Compendium de Phytotherapie, APB, 249, 1986

Specific references

13. Brophy J.J., Lassak E.V., Melaleuca leucadendra L. leaf oil: two phenylpropanoid chemotypes, Flavour Fragrance J., *3*, 43-46, 1988
14. Joseph J. Brophy, Erich V. Lassak, steam volatile leaf oils of some Melaleuca species from Western Australia, Flavour and Fragrance Journal, Vol. 7, 27-31, 1992
15. Lowry J.B., A new constituent of biogenetic, pharmacological and historical interest from Melaleuca cajeput oil, Nature, 241, 61-62, 1973
16. Motl O., Hodakova J., Ubik K., Composition of Vietnamese cajuput essential oil, Flavour Fragrance J., *5*, 39-42, 1990
17. Opdyke D.L.J., Food and Cosmetics Toxicology, *14* S, 701, 1976
18. Todorova M. & Ognyanov I., Composition of Vietnamese Essential oil from Melaleuca leucadendron L., Perfumer & Flavorist, *13*, 17-18
19. Recommendations concerning undesirable active principles, 3.8, 28th meeting Committee of Experts on Cosmetic Products, Rome, 3-7 November 1997, Council of Europe
20. BPC '73
21. Ned. F. 6
22. Ph. Esp.

Melaleuca viridiflora

Botanical name[1]	*Melaleuca viridiflora* Soland. ex Gaertn.
Botanical synonyms[2]	*Melaleuca leucadendron* L. var. *viridiflora* Gaertn.
Botanical family	Myrtaceae
Common name	Niaouli (English)
	Niaouli (Dutch)
	Niaouli (French)
	Niaouli (German)
	Niaouli (Italian)
	Niaouli (Norwegian)
	Niaouli (Spanish)
EU INCI name	-
CTFA INCI name	-

CAS number	8014-68-4 (essential oil)
EINECS number	
Parts used	Fresh leaves

Important constituents including active principles[3, 4, 8, 15]

- Essential oil (up to 2.6%)[3]:
  (Monoterpenes: α-pinene, α-thuyene, limonene, dipentene, π-cimene, sabinene, Δ³-carene, myrcene, phellandrene, α-humulene, β-selinene, α-terpineol, terpineol acetate and butyrate, cineole (up to 60%)[3]
  Sesquiterpenes: β-cariophyllene, cadinenes, nerolidol, linalool, viridoflorol, sesquiterpenol
  Aldehydes: benzaldehyde, butyraldehyde, isovalerianic aldehyde)

Preparation	Essential oil (Oil of Niaouli)
	Note: "Gomenol" is the Niaouli essential oil purified from aldehydes
Manufacturing process	Distillation of the fresh leaves
Examples of specifications[4]	Specific gravity at 15°C: 0.910-0.929
	Specific optical rotation: +0°42' to -3°34'
	Refractive index at 20°: 1.465 to 1.472
	Acid number: up to 2
	Ester number: 2 to 9
	Cineole content: 50 to 60%
	Solubility: soluble in about 1 vol. of 80% alcohol

Intended cosmetic effects and used concentration in cosmetic products

Tonic, deodorant, purifying; fragrance
Up to 0.3% in soaps and detergents, deodorants
Up to 10% in sport massage oils and liniments
Up to 0.1% in creams and lotions for atonic, impure skin

Other possible effects[8]

Granulation-promoting agent, antiseptic, hyperemic, analgesic, insect repellent

Main toxicological data[13]

(Eucalyptol or 1,8-cineole or p-cineole)
LD_{50} oral in rats: 2480 mg/kg
LD_{50} dermal in rabbits: >5 000mg/kg
Primary skin irritation: Applied undiluted to intact or abraded rabbit skin for 24 hr under occlusion it was not irritating.
Applied at 16% in petrolatum it produced no irritant effects after 48-hour closed-patch test in 25 human subjects
Sensitisation: No sensitisation effect when tested at 16% in petrolatum in 25 human subjects.

Has been studied sub-chronically in rats and mice; a NOEL of 300 mg/kg bw has been established. Eucalyptol has been found non-mutagenic in different systems.[16]

Databases used

CA Search 1967-95, Medline 1966-95, Embase 1974-95, Reg. Tox. Eff. Chem. Sub.

Keywords

Melaleuca viridiflora, Niaouli

Evaluation and remarks

Cat. A

General references

1. Index Kewensis, Clarendon Press
2. Penso G., Index Plantarum Medicinalium Totius Mundi Eorumque Synonymorum, OEMF, 1983
3. Fenaroli G., Sostanze Aromatiche Naturali, Hoepli ed., 785-787, 1963
4. Guenther E., The Essential oils, D. Van Nostrand, *4*, 535-539,1958
5. Martindale 31st ed., The Royal Pharmaceutical Society, 1996
6. Monograph Niaouli aetheroleum, Bundesanzeiger, No. 162 (Oct. 29, through Le monografie tedesche, Studio Edizioni, *2*, 1994
7. Proserpio G., Martelli A., Patri G.F., Elementi di fitocosmesi, Sepem, 1982
8. Paris R.R., Moyse H., Matière Médicale, Masson ed., *2*, 447, 1981
9. Van Hellemont J., Compendium de Phytotherapie, APB, 249, 1986

Specific references

10. Beylier M.F., Bacteriostatic activity of some Australian essential Oils, Perfum. Flavor., *4*, 23-26, 1979
11. De Medici D., Pieretti S., Salvatore G., Nicoletti M., Rasoanaivo P., Chemical analysis of essential oils of malgasy medicinal plant

by gas chromatography and NMR spectroscopy, Flavour Fragrance J., 7, 1992

12. Ministero della Guerra Italiano, Manuale dei medicamenti, Istituto Poligrafico dello Stato, *1*, 454 - 455,1934

13. Opdyke D.L.J., Food and Cosm. Toxicology, *13*, 105 - 108, 1975

14. Ramanoelina A.R.P., Viano J., Bianchini J.P., Gaydou E. M., Occurence of Various Chemotypes in Niaouli (*Melaleuca quinquenervia*) Essential Oils from Madagascar Using Multivariate Statistical Analysis, J. Agric. Food Chem, *42*, 1177-1182, 1994

15. Ramanoelina A.R.P., Viano J., Bianchini J.P. and Gaydou E. M., Andriantsiferana M., Chemical Composition of Niaouli Essential Oils from Madagascar, J. Essent. Oil Res., *4*, 657-658, 1992

16. Recommendations concerning undesirable active principles, 3.8, 28th Meeting Committee of Experts on Cosmetic Products, Rome, 3-7 November 1997, Council of Europe

17. Ph. B. V

18. Ned. F. 8

19. Ph. Fr. X

20. FU IX

Melilotus officinalis

Botanical name[1]	*Melilotus officinalis* Lam.
Botanical synonyms[1,2]	*Melilotus altissima* Thull., *Melilotus officinalis* (L.) Pallas
Botanical family	Fabaceae
Common names	Sweet clover (English)
	Akkerhoningklaver (Dutch)
	Rohtomesikkä (Finnish)
	Melilot (French)
	Steinklee (German)
	Meliloto (Italian)
	Legesteinkløver (Norwegian)
	Meliloto (Spanish)
	Sötväppling (Swedish)
EU INCI name[3]	*Melilotus officinalis*
CTFA INCI name[4]	Sweet clover (*Melilotus officinalis*) extract

CAS number	84082-81-5
EINECS number	282-028-5
Parts used	Flowered tops

Important constituents including active principles[13,15]
- Essential oil (up to 0.01%)[15]:
- Coumarins (coumarin 0.9%[15], melilotine 0.2%[34], melilotoside, scopoletine, umbelliferone)
- Flavonoids (quercetin, kaempferol) and isoflavonolds (medicarpin)[26]
- Tannins
- Saponins (melilotogenine[28], azukisaponine V, soyasapogenol B and E[30]
- Phenol acids[19,20] (o-hydroxycoumaric, π- and o-coumaric, melilotic, sinapic and ferulic acids)
- Hydrocarbons (limonene, nonadecan, heneicosan)
- Alcohols (2-phenylethanol)
- Choline
- Allantoin
- Resin
- Mucilages

Preparation
1) Dry hydroalcoholic extract E/D = 1:6[18]
2) Fluid hydroalcoholic extract E/D = 3:1[18]

3) Glycolic extract E/D = 4:1[18.]

4) Sweet clover extract[9.]

Manufacturing process Percolation with hydroalcoholic solution (60-70%) and concentration under vacuum to dryness
Percolation with hydroalcoholic solution (25-30%) and concentration under vacuum to final E/D ratio 3:1
Percolation with propylene glycol 45% to final E/D ratio 4:1
Obtained by extracting with water, ethanol, 1,3-butylene glycol, propylene glycol or a mixture of these solvents from the flower, leaf or flower and leaf

Examples of specifications 1) 2) 3) TLC-examination of coumarins
4) Heavy metals: not more than 20 ppm
Arsenic: not more than 2 ppm

Intended cosmetic effects and used concentration in cosmetic products
Soothing, astringent, refreshing

Other possible effects Capillary blood flow promoting agent[27.], anti-inflammatory, anti-oedema[21.], veinous astringent (haemorrhoids), analgesic, granulation-promoting agent, antimicrobial

Main toxicological data (fluid extract)[18.]
LD_{50} oral in rats and in mice: >50ml/kg
LD_{50} i.v. in rats and in mice: > 30 ml/kg
LD_{50} i.p. in rats: 1mg/kg
Mutagenicity (Ames test): negative
Alopecia due to dicoumarol was pointed out

(coumarin or 1,2-benzopyrone)[35.]
is carcinogenic in rodents, inducing liver tumours. It is mutagenic in a number of *in vitro* systems.[40.]

(quercetin, rutin)
Quercetin has been tested for carcinogenicity in a number of animal species and through several administration routes. An increased incidence of tumours has been observed in only one experiment in rats fed quercetin, whereas several other experiments using the same or higher doses did not provide any evidence of carcinogenic effects.
Rutin (the 3-rhamnoglucoside of quercetin) was tested in rats and hamsters with no evidence of carcinogenicity.

The *in vitro* pattern of genotoxicity of quercetin for different genetic endpoints is subject to a variety of factors such as pH, antioxidants, metabolism and nitrosation, whose role in each test system remains unclear, but evidence of *in vivo* mutagenicity of quercetin is still lacking.
Quercetin and other flavonoids have also been reported to have a number of positive effects including eicosanoid biosynthesis modification, protection of low-density lipoproteins from oxidation, pre-

vention of platelet aggregation and promotion of relation of cardiovascular smooth muscle.[41]

Databases used

CA Search 1967-96, Medline 1966-96, Embase 1974-96, Reg. Tox. Eff. Chem. Sub., IPA, Napralert, Toxline, Cosmet Database

Keywords

Melilotus officinalis

Evaluation and remarks

Cat. C

General references

1. Index Kewensis, Clarendon Press
2. Penso G., Index Plantarum Medicinalium Totius Mundi Eorumque Synonymorum, OEMF, 1983
3. European Commission Decision 96/335/EC of 8 May 1996, Official Journal of the European Community No. L132 of 1 June 1996
4. International Cosmetic Ingredient Dictionary 6th ed., CTFA, 2, 1995
5. Comprehensive Licensing Standards of Cosmetics by Category-4- 362, Yakuji Nippo, Ltd., 1989
6. Council of Europe, Flavouring substances and natural sources of flavourings, 3rd ed., (279 N3), Maisonneuve, 1981
7. Fenaroli G., Le sostanze aromatiche, Hoepli ed., 730-731, 1963
8. Grieve M., A modern herbal, Barnes & Noble Books, 2, 525-527, 1996
9. Japanese Cosmetic Ingredients Codex, ed. Yakuji Nippo LTD., 863, 1993
10. Martindale 31st ed., The Royal Pharmaceutical Society, 1996
11. Merck Index 12th ed., Merck & Co. Inc., 1996
12. Monograph Meliloti herba, Bundesanzeiger, No. 50 (Mar 13, 1986) and No. (Mar 13, 1990) through Le monografie tedesche, Studio Edizioni, 2, 1994
13. Paris R.R., Moyse H., Matière Médicale 2nd ed., Masson, 2, 391-392, 1981
14. Proserpio G., Martelli A., Patri G.F., Elementi di fitocosmesi, Sepem, 2, 1982
15. Van Hellemont J., Compendium de Phytotherapie, APB, 250-251, 1986
16. Wichtl M., Teedrogen, WVG, 470- 472, 1989

Specific references

17. Akras, Product specification
18. Austrian delegation Data Sheets, November 1995 and April 1996
19. Dombrowicz E., Swiatek L., Guryn R., Zadernowski R., Phenolic acids in herb Melilotus officinalis, Pharmazie 46, 156-157, 1991
20. Foldi-Borcsok E., Bedall F.K., Rahlfs V.W., Die antiphlogistische und odemhemmende Wirkung von Cumarin aus Melilotus officinalis, Arzneim.- Forsch.(Drug Res.) 21, 2025-2030, 1971
21. Hagers, Handbuch der Pharmazeutischen Praxis, Springer-Verlag, Auflage, 4. Bd., Chemikalien und Drogen CI-G, 755-757, 1973

22. Hagers, Handbuch der Pharmazeutischen Praxis, Springer-Verlag, Auflage, 5. Band, 755-758
23. Hoppe H. A., Drogenkunde, W. de Gruyter., 8. Auflage, 700-701, 1975
24. Hoppe H. A., Drogenkunde, W. de Gruyter, 180-181, 1981
25. Ingham J.L., Phytoalexin production by high- and low- coumarin cultivars of Melilotus alba and Melilotus officinalis, Can.J.Bot., *56*, 2230-2233, 1978
26. Kovàch A.G.B., Hamar J., Dora O., Marton I., Kunos G., Kun E., Die Wirkung von Cumarin aus Melilotus officinalis am Kreislauf des Hundes, Arzneim.- Forsch.(Drug Res.) *20*, 1630-1633, 1970
27. Kang S.S., Woo W.S., J. Nat. Prod., *51*, 335-338, 1988
28. Kang S.S., Lee Y.S., Lee E.B., Saengyak Hakhoechi, *18*, 89-93, 1987
29. Kang S.S., Lim C. H., Lee E.B., Arch. Pharmacol. Res. *10*, 9-13, 1987
30. Lebensmitteluntersuchung und- forschung, *190*, ISS 5, 425-428, 1990
31. Nater J.P., De Groot A.C., Unwanted effects of cosmetics and drugs used in dermatology, Excerpta Medica, 316,319, 1983
32. Nater J.P., De Groot A.C., Unwanted effects of cosmetics and drugs used in dermatology, Elsevier, 2nd ed., 383, 386, 1994
33. Melilotus officinalis L., C.E. 279, Comitato per lo Studio delle Bevande Alcoliche Aromatizzate, Torino, 1971
34. Opdyke D.L.J., Food and Cosm. Toxicology, *12*, 385- 405, 1974
35. Plantapharm, Fax vom, 16.11.1995
36. Richardson M.L., Gangoli S., the Dictionary of Substances and their Effects, Royal Society of Chemistry, 1992
37. Steinegger E., Hansel R., Lehrburch der Pharmakognosie, 3. Auflage, 1972, 5. Auflage, 690, 1981
38. Teuscher E., Lindequist U., Biogene Gifte, Akademic, 229, 1988
39. Wagner H., Bladt S., Zgainski E.M., Drogenanalyse, Springer, Dunnschichchromatographische Analyse von Arzneidrogen, S 156
40. Recommandations concerning undesirable active principles, 3.4, 28th meeting Committee of Experts on Cosmetic Products, Rome, 3-7 November 1997, Council of Europe.
41. Recommandations concerning undesirable active principles, 3.16, 28th meeting Committee of Experts on Cosmetic Products, Rome, 3-7 November 1997, Council of Europe.

Mimosa tenuiflora

Botanical name[1]	*Mimosa tenuiflora* (Willd.) Poir.
Botanical synonyms[1,4]	*Mimosa cabrera* Karst.
Botanical family	Mimosaceae
Common names	Tepescohuite (English)
	Mimosa (Finnish)
	Arbre de Peau (French)
	Mimosa (Norwegian)
	Mimosa (Spanish)
EU INCI name[2]	*Mimosa tenuiflora*
CTFA INCI name[3]	*Mimosa tenuiflora* leaf extract
	Mimosa tenuiflora bark extract

CAS number	93685-96-2
EINECS number	297-646-0
Parts used	Bark

Important constituents including active principles
- Triterpene saponins (mimonosides A, B and C)
- Steroid saponins as glycopyranosides and genins (lupeol, campesterol, stigmasterol, β-sitosterol)[5]
- Calcium oxalate
- Flavonoids
- Mineral salts
- Chalcones (kukulkanins A and B)[8]
- Starch
- Tannins (tannic acid, 4-ethyl-gallic acid)
- Alkaloids (indoleamine and methyltryptamine derivatives)

Preparation Hydroalcoholic extract E/D = 1:20

Manufacturing process[9] Percolation with a mixture of water and propylene glycol

Examples of specifications[9] pH: 5- 6.5
Propylene Glycol: 30%
Tannins: 0.13%
Flavonoids (calculated as rutin): 0.1- 0.12%

Intended cosmetic effects and used concentration in cosmetic products
Smoothing, soothing, protective, purifying
Up to 2% in products for chapped skin and lips, pre- and after-sun

products, detergents. Anti-ageing products[14], hair lotion, mouth-washes and toothpastes

Other possible effects

Anti-inflammatory, antimicrobial[10], granulation-promoting agent[12]., burns and UV erythema treatment[6,7], inhibitor of collagenase, elastase, hyaluronidase

Main toxicological data[9]

Primary skin irritation on rabbits: non-irritant
Acute eye irritation on rabbits: weakly irritant
Mutagenicity on Drosophila melanogaster: weakly mutagenic[13]

Databases used

CA Search 1967-95, Medline, 1966-95, Embase 1974-95, Reg. Tox. Eff. Chem. Sub.

Keywords

Mimosa tenuiflora, Tepescohuite, Tepezcohuite

Evaluation and remarks

Cat. B

General references

1. Index Kewensis, Clarendon Press
2. European Commission Decision 96/335/EC of 8 May 1996, Official Journal of the European Community No. L132 of 1 June 1996
3. International Cosmetic Ingredient Dictionary 6th ed. CTFA, *1*, 1995
4. Penso G., Index Plantarum Medicinalium Totius Mundi Eorumque Synonymorum, OEMF, 1983

Specific references

5. Anton R., Jiang Y., Weniger B. et al., Phamacognosy of Mimosa tenuiflora (Willd.) Poiret, Journal of Ethnopharmacology, *38*, 153-157, 1993
6. Cipriani C., Gelati G., Cozzani E., Effetti del Tepescohuite nei processi di cicatrizzazione, G. Ital. Dermatol. Venereol. *127*, 9, 447- 451,1992
7. Cipriani C., Gelati G., Cozzani E., Effetti del Tepescohuite nelle lesioni causate da raggi UV, G. Ital. Dermatol. Venereol. *128*, 1-2, 1-4, 1993
8. Dominguez X.A., Garcia S.G., et al., Kukulkanins A and B, new chalcones from Mimosa tenuiflora, Journal of Natural Products *52*, 4, 1989
9. Le Tepezcohuite le conquistador de la beauté, Parfums, cosmétiques, aromes *90*, 93-94, 1989
10. Lozoya X., Navarro V., Arnason J.T., Kourany E., Experimental evaluation of *Mimosa tenuiflora* (Willd.) Poir. (Tepescohuite). I.- screening of the antimicrobial properties of bark extract, Archiv. Invest. Méd. (Méx.), *20*, 87-93, 1989
11. Meckes-Lozoya M., Lozoya X., Gonzalez J.L., Propiedades Farmacològicas in vitro de algunos extractos de *Mimosa tenuiflora* (tepescohuite), Archiv. Invest. Méd. (Méx.), *21*, 163-169, 1990
12. Palacios C., Reyes R.E. et al, Efectos cicatrizante, antibacteriano y antimicótico del tepescohuite en animales de experimentación, Rev. Invest. Clin. *43*, 205-210, 1991

13. Pimentel A.E., Cruces M.P-, Zimmering S., Evaluation of the mutagenic potential of *tepezcohuite* in the Drosophila wing spot test, Mutation Research, *264*, 115-116, 1991
14. Proprietà ed impieghi cosmetici della Mimosa tenuiflora, COSNDG, *94*, 1991
15. Villarreal M.L., Alonso D., Melesio G, Cytotoxic activity of some Mexican plants used in traditional medicine, Fitoterapia Volume LXIII, N 6, 1992

Myristica fragrans

Botanical name[1]	*Myristica fragrans* Houtt.
Botanical synonyms[2]	*Myristica moschata* Thunb., *Myristica officinalis* L.
Botanical family	Myristicaceae
Common names	Nutmeg (English)
	Nootmuscaat (Dutch)
	Muskotti (Finnish)
	Noix muscade (French)
	Muskatnuss (German)
	Noce moscata (Italian)
	Muskat (Norwegian)
	Nuez moscada (Spanish)
	Muskot (Swedish)
EU INCI name[3]	*Myristica fragrans*
CTFA INCI name[4]	Nutmeg (*Myristica fragrans*) extract
	Nutmeg (*Myristica fragrans*) oil

CAS number	84082-68-8
	8008-45-5 (essential oil)
EINECS number	282-013-3
Parts used	Seeds (nutmeg) and arils (mace)

Important constituents including active principles[10]

- Essential oil (7-16%)

  Monoterpenes (α- and β-pinene, camphene, dipentene, π-cymene, α-thujene, γ-terpinene, sabinene, cineole, linalool, geraniol, terpinen-4-ol, borneol, α-terpineol and esters)

  Sesquiterpenes (α- cubebene, α-copaene, α-bergamoptene, β-cariophyllene, β- bisabolene, δ-cadinene, trans and cis-sabinene, cis-piperitol, dehydrodiisoeugenol, cis-p-menth-2-enol)

  Phenol ethers (myristicin (4-8%)[10], elemicin, isoelemicin, safrole, isosafrole, eugenol, isoeugenol, methyleugenol, methyliso-eugenol, methoxyeugenol)

- Triglycerides (lauric, tridecanoic, palmitic, stearic and myristic acids)
- Organic acids (formic, acetic, butyric, caprylic acid and their esters)
- Polyphenols (catechins, proanthocyanidins, lignans, neolignans)
- Saponins
- Aldehydes (citronellal, decanal)
- Resorcinols (malabaricone B and C)

– Carotenoids
– Unsaponifiable matter
– Phytosterols
– Starch (30%)[10]
– Tannins
– Proteins (6%)[10.]

Preparation 1) Essential oil

Manufacturing process 1) Steam distillation of crushed seeds

Examples of specifications 1)[9.] Specific gravity at 25°/25°: 0.880 to 0.913
Specific optical rotation: +7° 53' to +22° 10'
Refractive index at 20°: 1.4776 to 1.4861
Evaporation residue: 0.3 to 2.1%
Solubility at 20°: soluble in 1 to 2.5 vol. and more of 90% alcohol

Intended cosmetic effects and used concentration in cosmetic products
Tonic, purifying; flavour; fragrance
Up to 0.3% in toothpastes
Up to 0.2% in creams, lotions, detergents, soaps
Concentration limited in oils and emulsions for sports massage

Other possible effects[10, 16.] Anti-inflammatory and antirheumatic (myristicin)[20.], platelet aggregation inhibitor (eugenol, isoeugenol)[23.], analgesic, antimicrobial[27.], vasodilator

Main toxicological data (Elemicin)
Studies on the carcinogenicity of elemicin were negative, but those on the 1-hydroxy-metabolite were positive. No mutagenicity data are available, but the UDS assay of elemicin was positive[30.].

(Eucalyptol or 1,8-cineole or p-cineole)
has been studied sub-chronically in rats and mice; a NOEL of 300 mg/kg bw has been established. Eucalyptol has been found non-mutagenic in different systems[30.]

(Methyleugenol)
Methyleugenol and its 1-hydroxy-metabolite have been shown to be mutagenic in a number of system and to form liver DNA adducts in mice. It also increased hepatic tumour incidence in pre-weaned mice[30.]

(Myristicin)
Oleoresins from nutmeg fruits were found to be mutagenic in two Salmonella strains. Myristicin forms liver DNA adducts. Metabolism of myristicin yields 1-hydroxymyristicin, which is thought to be a proximate carcinogen[30.]

(Safrole)
Safrole is a weak liver carcinogen in rats and mice and is also a transplacental carcinogen in mice. Safrole has been found to be mutagenic in a number of systems[30.]

(Isosafrole)
Isosafrole is a weak liver carcinogen in rodents, but is non-mutagenic and has a low activity in forming liver DNA adducts.
Assumingthat hepatocarcinogenicity of isosafrole is associated with hepatic enzyme action a no effect level could be established: 50 mg/kg bw per day

Databases used

CA Search 1967-95, Medline, 1966-95, Embase 1974-95, Reg. Tox. Eff. Chem. Sub., IPA, Napralert, Toxline, Cosmet

Keywords

Myristica fragrans, Nutmeg

Evaluation and remarks

Cat. C

General references

1. Index Kewensis, Clarendon Press
2. Penso G., Index Plantarum Medicinalium Totius Mundi Eorumque Synonymorum, OEMF, 1983
3. European Commission Decision 96/335/EC of 8 May 1996, Official Journal of the European Community No. L132 of 1 June 1996
4. International Cosmetic Ingredient Dictionary 6th ed., CTFA, *1,* 1995
5. Council of Europe, Flavouring substances and natural sources of flavourings 3rd ed., Maisonneuve, (296 N2), 1981
6. Fenaroli G., Le sostanze aromatiche, Hoepli ed., 790-794, 1963
7. Flavouring Extract Manufacturers Association (Fema), Survey of flavouring ingredients usage levels, (No.2792, 2793), Food Technology, (286), *2,* 1965
8. Grieve M., A modern herbal, Barnes & Noble Books, 591-592, 1996
9. Guenther E., The Essential oils, D. Van Nostrand, *5,* 59-81, 1952
10. Leung A.Y., Foster S., Encyclopedia of common natural ingredients, Wiley & Son Publ., 385-388, 1996
11. Martindale 31st ed., The Royal Pharmaceutical Society, 1996
12. Merck Index 12th ed., Merck & Co. Inc., 1996
13. Monograph Myristicae semen - Myristicae arillus, Bundesanzeiger, n. (Sept 18, 1986) through Le monografie tedesche, Studio Edizioni, 1994
14. Paris R.R., Moyse H., Matière Médicale 2nd ed., Masson, *2,* 169-170, 1981
15. Proserpio G., Martelli A., Patri G.F., Elementi di fitocosmesi, Sepem, *2,* 1983
16. Van Hellemont J., Compendium de Phytotherapie, APB, 258-259, 1986

Specific references

17. Akras Product specification
18. Futrell J.M., Rietschel R.L., CUTIS 52, 288-290, 1988
19. Hada S., Hattori M. et al., New Neolignans and Lignans from the Aril of Myristica fragrans, Phytochemistry, *27,* 2, 563-568, 1988

20. Handa S.S., Chawla A.S., Sharma A.K., Plants with Anti-inflammatory activity, Fitoterapia, *63*, 1, 3-31, 1992
21. Hagers, Handbuch der Pharmazeutischen Praxis, Springer, 5. Auflage, Bd. 5 Drogen, 863-894 , 1993
22. Hagers, Handbuch der Pharmazeutischen Praxis, Springer Verlag, 5. Auflage, Bd. 3 Gifte, 853 f, 1993
23. Janssens J., Laekeman G.M. et al., Nutmeg oil: Identification and Quantitation of its Most Active Constituents as Inhibitors of Platelet Aggregation, Journal of Ethnopharmacology, *29*, 179-188, 1990
24. Lawrence B.M., Perf & Flav., *15*, 66, 1990
25. Opdyke D.L. J., Food and Cosmetics Toxicology, *14*, 6, 631-633, 1976
26. Opdyke D.L.J., Food and Cosmetics Toxicology, *17*, 2s, 851-852, 1979
27. Orabi K., Mossa J.S., El-Feraly F.S., Isolation and Characterisation of two Antimicrobial Agents from mace (*Myristica fragrans*)
28. Pino J.A., Borges P., Mollinedo B., Nota. Aceite esencial de nuez moscada (*Myristica fragrans* H.): Obtención y caracterización de su composición química, Rev. Agroquím. Tecnol. Aliment., *31*, 3, 411-416, 1991
29. Wirth, Gloxhuber, Toxikologie, G.Thieme Verlag, 409, 1994
30. Recommendations concerning undesirable active principles, 3.5, 3.8, 3.11, 3.13, 3.18, 28th meeting Committee of Experts on Cosmetic Products, Rome, 3-7 November 1997, Council of Europe
31. Ph. B. IV
32. Ph. Helv VII
33. BP '88
34. OAB '90
35. USP XXI
36. Belg VI

Nasturtium officinale

Botanical name[1]	*Nasturtium officinale* R. Br.
Botanical synonyms[2]	*Nasturtium fontanum* Aschers, *Roripa nasturtium* Beck, *Roripa nasturtium* Rusby, *Roripa nasturtium-aquaticum* Hay, *Sisymbrium nasturtium* Thunb.)
Botanical family	Brassicaceae
Common names	Watercress (English)
	Witte waterkers (Dutch)
	Isovesikrassi (Finnish)
	Cresson de fontaine (French)
	Brunnenkresse (German)
	Crescione (Italian)
	Engelsk karse (Norwegian)
	Berro de agua (Spanish)
	Källkrasse (Swedish)
EU INCI name[3]	*Nasturtium officinale*
CTFA INCI name[4]	Water cress (*Nasturtium officinale*) extract

CAS number	84775-70-2
EINECS number	283-899-4
Parts used	Aerial part

Important constituents including active principles[13]

- Essential oil (up to 0.066%)[8]
- Glucosinolates (2-phenylethylglucosinolate, 7-methylthioeptilglucosinolate, 8-methylthioottilglucosinolate). By autolysis forming mainly phenylethylisothiocyanate.
- Hydrogen cyanide[20]
- Flavonoids
- Sugars
- Carotenoids
- Vitamins (B_1, B_2, C, E, PP)
- Mineral salts (iodine, iron, calcium, phosphorus)
- Triglycerides

Preparation
1) Hydroglycolic extract[19]
2) Watercress extract[6]

Manufacturing process	1)[19] Percolation with propylene glycol 50% to final E/D ratio 1:1
	2)[6] Extraction of the leaves and stems or herb with purified water, ethanol, propylene glycol, 1,3-butylene glycol or the mixture of these.

Examples of specifications

1)[19] pH: 5.9 to 6.9
Relative density at 20°C: 1.035 to 1.045
Refractive index at 20°C: 1.388 to 1.392
Dry residue: 0.10 to 60%
Heavy metals: < 40 ppm

2)[6] Heavy metals: not more than 10 ppm
Arsenic: not more than 1 ppm

Intended cosmetic effects and used concentration in cosmetic products

Tonic, lightening, purifying
Up to 7% in emulsions, cleaning lotion, gels and detergents for oily and impure skin
Up to 12% in lotions, detergents and conditioners for oily scalp and hair treatment
Hair loss treatment (traditional use)

Other possible effects

Anti-eczema, whitening

Main toxicological data

(Extract)
LD_{50} i.p. in rat: 1000 mg/kg [(RTECS) 18]
Primary skin irritation on rabbits: non-irritant[21]
Acute eye irritation on rabbits: non-irritant[21]

(Hydrogen cyanide)[20]
LD_{50} oral in mice: 3.7 mg/kg b.w.

Databases used

CA Search 1967-97, Medline 1966-97, Embase 1974-97, Ref. Tox. Eff. Chem. Sub., Biosis, Toxline, Kosmet

Keywords

Nasturtium officinale, Roripa nasturtium, Watercress

Evaluation and remarks

Cat. A (hydroalcoholic extract; watercress extract)

Taken in strong doses and internally, glucosinolates, which are generally regarded as slightly rubefacient, may cause hypofunctioning of the thyroid.

General references

1. Index Kewensis, Clarendon Press
2. Penso G., Index Plantarum Medicinalium Totius Mundi Eorumque Synonymorum, OEMF, 1983
3. European Commission Decision 96/335/EC of 8 May 1996, Official Journal of the European Community No. L132 of 1 June 1996
4. International Cosmetic Ingredient Dictionary 6th ed., CTFA, 1995
5. Benigni R., Capra C., Cattorini P.E., Piante Medicinali chimica farmacologia e terapia, Inverni & Della Beffa, *2,* 974-977, 1964
6. Comprehensive Licensing Standards of Cosmetics by Category, Yakuji Nippo Ltd., *2,* 431, 1987

7. Council of Europe, Flavouring substances and natural sources of flavourings 3rd ed. Maisonneuve, (301 N1), 1981
8. Fenaroli G., Sostanze Aromatiche Naturali, Hoepli, 777-778, 1963
9. Grieve M., A modern herbal, Barnes & Noble Books, 845, 1996
10. Guenther E., The Essential oils, D. Van Nostrand, 1952
11. The Japanese Cosmetic Ingredients Codex, ed. Yakuji Nippo Ltd., 939, 1993
12. Paris R.R., Moyse H., Matière Médicale, Masson 2nd ed., *2*, 219, 1981
13. Proserpio G., Martelli A., Patri G.F., Elementi di fitocosmesi, Sepem, 509, 2, 1983
14. Van Hellemont J., Compendium de Phytotherapie, APB, 261-262, 1986
15. Wichtl M., Teedrogen, WVG, 124-125, 1989
16. Ph.B.II

Specific references

17. Azuma S., Yada Y., Imokawa G., Tazaki S., Shinho T., Skin-lightening cosmetics containing plant extract and ascorbic acid or placenta extract, JP 08,208,451 [96,208,451], 13 Aug 1996
18. CE Data sheets Nov. 1996
19. Indena Product Specifications
20. Duke J., CRC Crit. Rev. Toxicol., *5*, 189, 1977
21. Indena's reports

Olea europaea (fruits)

Botanical name[1]	*Olea europaea* L.
Botanical synonyms[2]	*Olea sativa* Hoffsmeg et Link.
Botanical family	Oleaceae
Common names	Olive tree (English)
	Olijfboom (Dutch)
	Oliivi (Finnish)
	Olivier (French)
	Olbaum, Olivenbaum (German)
	Olivo (Italian)
	Oliventre (Norwegian)
	Olivo (Spanish)
	Olivträd (Swedish)
EU INCI name[3]	*Olea europaea*
CTFA INCI name[4]	1) Olive (*Olea europaea*) extract
	2) Olive (*Olea europaea*) oil unsaponifiables

CAS number	1) 84012-27-1
	2) 8001-25-0
EINECS number	1) 232-277-0
	2) 232-277-0
Parts used	Fruits

Important constituents including active principles

- Triglycerides (up to 20%)[12] (containing oleic 70-75%, palmitic 12-15%, linoleic 10% and linolenic acids)[12]
- Free fatty acids
- Flavonoids (cyanidin, luteolin, quercetin and apigenin glycosides)
- Secoiridoids (oleuropein and dimethyloleuropein)
- Phenol acids (p-coumaric, caffeic acid, tyrosol and hydroxytyrosol)
- Unsaponifiables (0.5-1.5%)15.:
  Hydrocarbons (squalene 75%)
  Triterpene alcohols (6.5-8.5%) (α- and β-amyrin, cycloarthenol, 24-methylcycloarthenol, erythriodiol, uvaol)
  Monoterpene alcohols (linalol and citronellol)
  Aliphatic alcohols (C18-C40, mainly C22-C30)
  Phytosterols (7-10%) (campesterol, stigmasterol, β-sitosterol)
  Vitamins (mainly E about 0.2%)
- Proteins (2%)[12]

Preparation	Unsaponifiables
Manufacturing process	Saponification and partition between butylalcohol and hexane
Examples of specifications	(Unsaponifiables)[19.]

Specific gravity at 20°C: 0.878-0.895
Refractive index at 10°C: 1.490-1.590
Solubility: soluble in vegetable and animal oils; partially soluble in mineral oil and synthetic esters.
OH number: 5-15
Acid number: max. 0.5
Iodine number: 275-295
Saponification number: max 5
Unsaponifiable: 97-99%

Intended cosmetic effects and used concentration in cosmetic products

(Oil)
Emollient, smoothing, soothing, refreshing for delicate skin
Up to 10% in oils, emulsions and lipogels. In sun products.

(Unsaponifiables)
Emollient, smoothing for dry and ageing skin, soothing, sunscreen, emulsifier
Up to 5% in pre- and after-sun products, hair conditioners, preparations for sensitive skin and swollen gums

Other possible effects

(Oil)
Traditional use in ointments for wounds, burns, dermatosis, stretch marks, breast firming, anti-inflammatory

(Unsaponifiables)
Anti-inflammatory, healing agent on wounds and burns, melanin biosynthesis activator

Main toxicological data

(Oil)
Adverse cutaneous reactions to topically applied olive oil are seldom reported.[18.]

(Oleuropein)[16.]
LD50 i.p. in mice: 1000 mg/kg body wt

Databases used

CA Search 1967-97, Medline 1966-97, Embase 1974-97, Ref. Tox. Eff. Chem. Sub., Toxline; Toxbio; Toxcas

Keywords

Olea europea, olive

Evaluation and remarks

Cat. A (unsaponifiables)

Unsaponifiables have many properties, notably as anti-inflammatories, without any apparent toxicity.

General references

1. Index Kewensis, Clarendon Press

2. Penso G., Index Plantarum Medicinalium Totius Mundi Eorumque Synonymorum, OEMF, 1983

3. European Commission Decision 96/335/EC of 8 May 1996, Official Journal of the European Community No. L132 of 1 June 1996
4. International Cosmetic Ingredient Dictionary 6th ed., CTFA, 1995
5. Benigni R., Capra C., Cattorini P.E., Piante Medicinali chimica farmacologia e terapia, Inverni & Della Beffa, 1012- 1022, 2, 1, 1964
6. Council of Europe, Flavouring substances and natural sources of flavourings 3rd ed. Maisonneuve, (309 N 1), 1981
7. Grieve M., A modern herbal, Barnes & Noble Books, 598-599, 1996
8. The Japanese Cosmetic Ingredients, second edition, Yakuji Nippo, LTD, 217-218, 1985
9. Martindale 31st ed., The Royal Pharmaceutical Society, 1996
10. Merck Index 12th ed., Merck & Co. Inc., 1996
11. Paris R.R., Moyse H., Matière Mèdicale, Masson ed., 3, 27-32, 1971
12. Proserpio G., Martelli A., Patri G.F., Elementi di fitocosmesi, Sepem, 2, 777-778, 1983
13. Van Hellemont J., Compendium de Phytotherapie, APB, 268-270, 1986

Specific references

14. Camurati F., Rizzolo A., Fedeli E. I componenti chimici delle parti anatomiche del frutto dell'Olea europea. Part.II: estratti alcolici, Riv. It. Sost. Grasse, 58, 541-547, 1981
15. Cravini S., Gli insaponificabili, Il prodotto chimico, 12-17, 1986
16. Hänsel R. et al (eds.), Hagers Handbuch der Pharmazeutischen Praxis, 5th ed. 1993
17. Hoppe, Drogenkunde, 8th ed., 1975
18. Kränke B., Komericki P. and Aberer W., Olive oil- contact sensitizer or irritant?, Contact Derm. 36, 1, 5-10, 1997
19. Massera A.M., Fedeli E., Proserpio G., Insaponificabile in toto da Olea europea, Rivista Italiana E.P.P.O.S. 60, 7, 414-421, 1978
20. Nater J.P., de Groot A.C., Unwanted effects of cosmetics and drugs used in dermatology, Elsevier Science Publishers B.V., 1985
21. Rovellini P., Cortesi N., Fedeli E., Analysis of flavonoids from Olea europea by HPLC-UV and HPLC-electrospray-MS, Rivista Italiana Sostanze Grasse, 74, 273-279, 1997
22. Zander, Pflanzennamen, 15 ed., 1994
23. Thorel Jean-Noël Brevet Cl. Λ 61 K 7/10, 1 DCC. 1992
24. Ph Eur.
25. DAB 10
26. OAB 90
27. Ph Helv VII
28. Ph Fr IX
29. Ph B V
30. Ned F 6

Olea europaea (leaves)

Botanical name[1]	*Olea europaea* L.
Botanical synonyms[2]	*Olea sativa* Hoffsmeg et Link.
Botanical family	Oleaceae
Common names	Olive tree (English)
	Olijfboom (Dutch)
	Oliivi (Finnish)
	Olivier (French)
	Olbaum, Olivenbaum (German)
	Olivo (Italian)
	Oliventre (Norwegian)
	Olivo (Spanish)
	Olivträd (Swedish)
EU INCI name[3]	*Olea europaea*
CTFA INCI name[4]	Olive (*Olea europaea*) leaf extract

CAS number	84012-27-1
EINECS number	232-277-0
Parts used	Leaves

Important constituents including active principles

- Sesquiterpenes (aromadendrene, eudesmin)
- Triterpenes (2-4%) (oleanolic acid up to 3%[12], homoolestranol, maslinic acid, erythrodiol, uvaol)
- Flavonoids (luteolin-4-glucoside, luteolin, olivin, rutin, apigenin)
- Secoiridoids (4-7%) (oleuropeine 6-9%[16], demethyloleuropeine, excelsioside, verbascoside, oleoside, oleosidedimethylester, oleoside-11-methylether, ligstroside, ligustaloside B, morroniside, oleacein)
- Lignans (olivyl-4-glucoside, acetoxypinoresinol, cyclolivyle)
- Phytosterols (campesterol, stigmasterol, β-sitosterol)
- Polyalcohol (mannitol)
- Hydrocarbons C_{30}-C_{33} (squalene)
- Triglycerides
- Long chain esthers
- Dimethylbenzoquinone (0.02%)[16]
- α-Hydroxyacids (lactic, malic, glycolic, tartaric acids)
- Tannins
- Alkaloids (traces) (cinchonin, cinchonidin, dihydrocinchonine)

Preparation

Fluid hydroalcoholic extract

Manufacturing process

Percolation with alcohol 20% and concentration under vacuum to final E/D ratio 1:1.

Examples of specifications -

Intended cosmetic effects and used concentration in cosmetic products

Skin tonic, astringent, soothing

Up to 10% in creams and lotions

Other possible effects

Anti-inflammatory, antiseptic, antioxidant[21.]

Main toxicological data

(Extract)[16.]

LD_{50} i.p. in mice: 1300 mg/kg body wt

(Oleuropein)[16.]

LD_{50} i.p. in mice: 1000 mg/kg body wt.

Databases used

CA Search 1967-97, Medline 1966-97, Embase 1974-97, Ref. Tox. Eff. Chem. Sub., Toxline; Toxbio; Toxcas

Keywords

Olea europea, olive

Evaluation and remarks

Cat. B (hydroalcoholic fluid extract)

A priori **not toxic, or only slightly toxic, but further information required.**

General references

1. Index Kewensis, Clarendon Press
2. Penso G., Index Plantarum Medicinalium Totius Mundi Eorumque Synonymorum, OEMF, 1983
3. European Commission Decision 96/335/EC of 8 May 1996, Official Journal of the European Community No. L132 of 1 June 1996
4. International Cosmetic Ingredient Dictionary 6th ed., CTFA, 1995
5. Benigni R., Capra C., Cattorini P.E., Piante Medicinali chimica farmacologia e terapia, Inverni & Della Beffa, 1012- 1022, 2, 1, 1964
6. Council of Europe, Flavouring substances and natural sources of flavourings 3rd ed. Maisonneuve, (309 N 2), 1981
7. Grieve M., A modern herbal, Barnes & Noble Books, 598-599, 1996
8. Martindale 31st ed., The Royal Pharmaceutical Society, 1996
9. Merck Index 12th ed., Merck & Co. Inc., 1996
10. Monographs Olivae folium, Bundesanzeiger , No. 11 (17 Jan. 1991), through Le monografie tedesche, Studio Edizioni, 2,1994
11. Paris R.R., Moyse H., Matière Médicale, Masson ed., 3, 27-32, 1971
12. Proserpio G., Martelli A., Patri G.F., Elementi di fitocosmesi, Sepem, 2, 511-512, 1983
13. Van Hellemont J., Compendium de Phytotherapie, APB, 268-270, 1986

Specific references

14. Cortesi N., Mosconi C., Fedeli E., Cromatografia liquida ad alta risoluzione nell'analisi di estratti fogliari di *Olea europea*, Rivista Italiana Sostanze Grasse, *61*, 549-557, 1984

15. De Nino A. et al., Direct Identification of Phenolic Glucosides from Olive Leaf Extracts by Atmospheric Pressure Ionisation Tandem Mass Spectrometry, Journal of Mass Spectrometry, *32*, 533-541, 1997

16. Hänsel R. et al (eds.), Hagers Handbuch der Pharmazeutischen Praxis, 5th ed. 1993

17. Hoppe, Drogenkunde, 8th ed., 1975

18. Le Tutour B., Guedon D., Antioxidantive Activities of Olea europea leaves and related phenolic compounds, Phytochemistry, *31*, 4, 1173-1178, 1992

19. NaterJ.P., de Groot A.C., Unwanted effects of cosmetics and drugs used in dermatology, Elsevier Science Publishers B.V., 1985

20. Rovesti P., Oil and extracts of olive leaves, the Indian oil and soap journal, *33*, 10, 276-284, 1968

21. Rovellini P., Cortesi N., Fedeli E., Analysis of flavonoids from Olea europea by HPLC-UV and HPLC-electrospray-MS, Rivista Italiana Sostanze Grasse, *74*, 273-279, 1997

22. Yamamoto A., Kang S., Dosui K., Antioxidants from olive extracts for food, cosmetic and pharmaceutical preparations, JP 09 78,061 [97 78,061], 25 Mar 1997

23. Zander, Pflanzennamen, 15 ed., 1994

24. Ph Eur.

25. DAB 10

26. OAB 90

27. Ph Helv VII

28. Ph Fr IX

29. Ph B V

30. Ned F 6

Passiflora incarnata

Botanical name[1]	*Passiflora incarnata* L.
Botanical synonyms	-
Botanical family	*Passifloraceae*
Common names	Passionflower (English)
	Passiekruid (Dutch)
	Kärsimyskukka (Finnish)
	Herbe de la passion (French)
	Passionblume (German)
	Passiflora (Italian)
	Pasjonsblomst (Norwegian)
	Pasionaria (Spanish)
	Passionsblomma (Swedish)
EU INCI name[2]	*Passiflora incarnata*
CTFA INCI name[3]	Passionflower (*Passiflora incarnata*) extract
	Passionflower (*Passiflora incarnata*) fruit extract

CAS number	84012-31-7 (extract)
	72968-47-9
EINECS number	277-142-7
Parts used	Twigs with flowers and fruits

Important constituents including active principles[7, 11, 14]

- Essential oil (hexanal, benzylalcohol, linalool, 2-phenylethylalcohol, 2-hydroxybenzoic acid methylester, carvone, trans anethole, eugenol, isoeugenol, β-ionone, α-bergamotol, phytol)[18]
- Flavonoids (1.5-2.2%)[14] (vitexin, isovitexin, isovitexin- 2"-O-β-glycoside, orientin, isoorientin, isoorientin- 2"-O-β-glycoside, quercetin, kaempferol, saponarin, saponaretin, rutin, apigenin and apigenin-glucoside, luteolin and luteolin-glucoside, schaftoside, isoschaftoside, vicenin, lucenin, swertisin)
- Indole alkaloids (harman, harmine, harmol, harmaline, harmalol) (up to 0.09%)[7]
- Cyanogenic glycoside (gynocardin) (traces)[10]
- Maltol (0.05%)[15], ethyl-maltol
- Phytosterols (β-sitosterol, stigmasterol)
- Sugars (raffinose and sucrose)
- Hydrocarbons (*n*-nonacosane)
- Fatty acids (palmitic and oleic acids)
- Gums

Preparation	Dry hydroalcoholic extract
Manufacturing process	Percolation with alcohol and concentration under vacuum to dryness
Examples of specifications[17]	Assay: 3.5-4.0 flavonoids as isovitexin Water (K. Fischer): not more than 6.0% Sulphated ash: not more than 20.0% Heavy metals: not more than 100 ppm pH (c=1, water): 4.0-6.0

Intended cosmetic effects and used concentration in cosmetic products
Soothing, smoothing, protective
Up to 2% in products for sensitive skin.
Bath preparations (traditional use)[7]

Other possible effects	(Flavonoids) Microcirculation protector, free radical scavenger, anti-irritant, antioxidant, purifying for acneic skin
Main toxicological data[20]	(Extract) [RTECS, 17] TDL_0 oral in rats: 440 mg/kg 7-170 preg LD_{50} oral in mice and rats: > 15 000 mg/kg LD_{50} i.p. in rats: 3510 mg/kg LD_{50} i.p. in mice: 3140 mg/kg LD_{50} subcutaneous in rats: > 10 000 mg/kg LD_{50} subcutaneous in mice: 8300 mg/kg Acute dermal irritation in rabbits: not irritant Acute eye irritation in rabbits: in progress

(maltol)[16]
LD_{50} i.p. in mice: 820 mg/kg

(ethylmaltol)[16]
LD_{50} i.p. in mice: 910 mg/kg

(quercetin, rutin)
Quercetin has been tested for carcinogenicity in a number of animal species and through several administration routes. An increased incidence of tumours has been observed in only one experiment in rats fed quercetin, whereas several other experiments using the same or higher doses did not provide any evidence of carcinogenic effects.
Rutin (the 3-rhamnoglucoside of quercetin) was tested in rats and hamsters with no evidence of carcinogenicity.

The *in vitro* pattern of genotoxicity of quercetin for different genetic endpoints is subject to a variety of factors such as pH, antioxidants, metabolism and nitrosation, whose role in each test system remains unclear, but evidence of *in vivo* mutagenicity of quercetin is still lacking.
Quercetin and other flavonoids have also been reported to have a number of positive effects including eicosanoid biosynthesis modification, protection of low-density lipoproteins from oxidation, prevention of platelet aggregation and promotion of relation of cardiovascular smooth muscle.[19]

Databases used   CA Search 1967-95, Medline, 1966-95, Embase 1974-95, Reg. Tox.
                        Eff. Chem. Sub

Keywords   *Passiflora incarnata*

Evaluation and remarks   **Cat. A**

General references
1. Index Kewensis, Clarendon Press
2. European Commission Decision 96/335/EC of 8 May 1996, Official Journal of the European Community No. L132 of 1 June 1996
3. International Cosmetic Ingredient Dictionary 6th ed., CTFA, *1*, 1995
4. Benigni R., Capra C., Cattorini P.E., Piante Medicinali chimica farmacologia e terapia, Inverni & Della Beffa, *2*, 1080-1085, 1964
5. Council of Europe, Flavouring substances and natural sources of flavourings (321,N3), 3rd ed., Maisonneuve, 1981
6. Grieve M., A modern herbal, Barnes & Noble Books, *2*, 618, 1996
7. Leung A.Y., Foster S., Encyclopedia of common natural ingredients, Wiley & Son Publ., 408-411, 1996
8. Martindale 31st ed., The Royal Pharmaceutical Society, 1996
9. Merck Index 12th ed., Merck & Co. Inc., 1996
10. Monograph Passiflorae herba, Bundesanzeiger, No. 223 (Nov. 30, 1985) No. 50 (Mar. 13,1990) through Le monografie tedesche, Studio Edizioni, 1994
11. Newall C., Anderson L., Phillipson J.D., Herbal Medicines a guide for health care professionals, The Pharmaceutical Press, 206-207, 1996
12. Paris R.R., Moyse H., Matière Médicale 2nd ed., Masson, *2*, 519, 1981
13. Proserpio G., Martelli A., Patri G.F., Elementi di fitocosmesi, Sepem, *2*, 1983
14. Van Hellemont J., Compendium de Phytotherapie, APB, 283-284, 1986
15. Wichtl M., Teedrogen, WVG, 362-364, 1989

Specific references
16. Aoyagin N., Kimura R., Murata T., Studies on Passiflora incarnata Dry extract. I. Isolation of Maltol and Pharmacological Action of Maltol and Ethyl Maltol, Chem. Pharm. Bull., 22, 1008-1013, 1974
17. Indena, Products specification
18. Buchbauer G., Jirovetz L., Volatile Constituents of the Essential Oil of Passiflora incarnata L., J. Essent. Oil Res., 4, 329-334, 1992
19. Recommendations concerning undesirable active principles, 3.16, 28th meeting, Committee of Experts on Cosmetic Products, Rome, 3-7 November 1997, Council of Europe.
20. Indena's reports
21. FU IX
22. Ph. Fr. X
23. Ph. Helv VII,
24. DAB X
25. BHP, '90

Plantago spp.

Botanical name[1]	*Plantago major* L., *Plantago lanceolata* L., (are the main species used)
Botanical synonyms for *Plantago major*[2]	
	P. asiatica DC., *P. crenata* Blanco, *P. erosa* Wall., *P. officinarum* Crantz, *P. hasskarlii* Decne., *P. incisa* Hassk., *P. loureiri* Roem et Schult., *P. media* Blanco
Botanical varieties of *Plantago major*[2] **used**	
	Plantago major L. var. *cruenta* Holuby
	Plantago major L. var. *asiatica* DC.
	Plantago major L. var. *densiuscula*
Other species used[16, 17]	*P. maritima, P. macorrhiza, P. coronopus, P. depressa, P. japonica, P. camischatica, P. serpervirens, P. montana, P. indica* L. (= *P. arenaria*), *P. cynops,* L., *P. alpina* L., *P. loeflingii, P. inflexa, P. rhodosperma, P. purshii, P. aristata, P. albicans* L., *P. crypsoides* Boiss, *P. notata* Lag, *P. crassifolia* Forsk , *P. cylindrica* Forsk.
Botanical family	Plantaginaceae

Common names for *Plantago major*

Large plantain	(English)
Grote Weegbree	(Dutch)
Piharatamo	(Finnish)
Grand plantain	(French)
Breitwegerich	(German)
Piantaggine	(Italian)
Groblad	(Norwegian)
Llantén mayor	(Spanish)
Groblad	(Swedish)

for *Plantago lanceolata*

Small plantain	(English)
Smalbladige Weegbree	(Dutch)
Heinäratamo	(Finnish)
Plantain lanceolé	(French)
Spitzwegerich	(German)
Piantaggine lanceolata	(Italian)
Smalkjempe	(Norwegian)
Llantén meyor	(Spanish)
Svartkämpe	(Swedish)

EU INCI names[3]	*Plantago major* (*P. major*)
	Plantago lanceolata (*P. lanceolata*)
CTFA INCI names[4]	Plantain (*Plantago major*) extract (*P. major*)
	Plantain (*Plantago lanceolata*) extract (*P. lanceolata*)

CAS number	84929-43-1 (*P. major*)
	85085-64-9 (*P. lanceolata*)
EINECS number	284-526-8 (*P. major*)
	285-388-1 (*P. lanceolata*)
Parts used	Aerial parts (leaves)

Important constituents including active principles[5, 13]

- Polysaccharides (6,5%)[14] (containing: rhamnogalacturonane, arabinogalactane, glucomannane, pectins 5%[12])
- Iridoids (aucubin up to 2,5%[14], catalpol up to 1,1%[14], melitoside, asperuloside, majoroside, geniposidic acid)
- Phenol acids (p-hydroxybenzoic, ferulic, coumaric, gentisic, protocathecic, chlorogenic acids, caffeic acid and its ester, plantamajoside)[19]
- Coumarins (esculetin)
- Flavonoids (apigenin, luteolin, scutellarein)
- Tannins 4%[12]
- Lactone (lolioside)
- Alkaloids (plantagonine, indicaine)
- Mineral salts (silicic acid > 1%)[14]

Preparation[5]	Hydroalcoholic fluid extract E/D = 1:1
Manufacturing process[5]	Percolation with alcohol 20% and concentration under vacuum to final E/D ratio 1:1
Examples of specifications	-

Intended cosmetic effects and used concentration in cosmetic products

Smoothing, soothing, moisturising, astringent, purifying
The fresh juice is traditionally used for insect bites and it is also used as soothing agent for the eye contour.

Other possible effects	Granulation-promoting agent, anti-inflammatory, antibacterial[19], haemostatic.
Main toxicological data	Reports of hypersensitivity associated with ingestion or inhalation of Plantago spp. containing products.
	Reports of hypersensitivity, respiratory responses and allergic reactions.
	(aucubin)
	LDL_0 on mice: 0.9 g/kg
	Administration of 80 mg/kg, 4 times a week, in mice did not effect serum enzyme level or chemical parameters.
Databases used	CA Search 1967-96, Medline 1966-96, Embase 1974-96, Ref. Tox. Eff. Chem, Sub., Excerpta Medica, Life Sciences, Cosmet, Biosis, Previews, Cancerlit, Toxline, Int. Pharm. Abstract
Keywords	*Plantago major, Plantago lanceolata*
Evaluation and remarks	**Cat. B**

General references

1. Index Kewensis, Clarendon Press
2. Penso G., Index Plantarum Medicinalium Totius Mundi Eorumque Synonymorum, OEMF, 1983
3. European Commission Decision 96/335/EC of 8 May 1996, Official Journal of the European Community No. L132 of 1 June 1996
4. International Cosmetic Ingredient Dictionary 6th ed., CTFA, *1*, 1995
5. Benigni R., Capra C., Cattorini P.E., Piante Medicinali chimica farmacologia e terapia, Inverni & Della Beffa, *2*, 1100-1103, 1964
6. Council of Europe, Flavouring substances and natural sources of flavourings 3rd ed., Maisonneuve, (352 N2), 1981
7. Grieve M., A modern herbal, Barnes & Noble Books, *2*, 640-642, 644, 1996
8. Martindale 31st ed., The Royal Pharmaceutical Society, 1996
9. Monograph Plantaginis lanceolatae herba, Bundesanzeiger, n. 223 (Nov 30, 1985) through Le monografie tedesche, Studio Edizioni, *2*, 1994
10. Newall C., Anderson L., Phillipson J.D., Herbal Medicines: a guide for health care professionals, The Pharmaceutical Press, 210-212, 1996
11. Paris R.R., Moyse H., Matière Médicale, Masson, *3*, 300, 1971
12. Proserpio G., Martelli A., Patri G.F., Elementi di fitocosmesi, Sepem, *2*, 818, 1982
13. Van Hellemont J., Compendium de Phytotherapie, APB, 299-301, 1986
14. Wichtl M., Teedrogen, WVG, 466-469, 1989

Specific references

15. Brautigam M., Franz G., Structural Features of *Plantago lanceolata* Mucilage, Planta Medica, 293-297, 1985
16. Hansel R. et al. Hrsg, Drogen, 221-222, 1994
17. Hoppe H. A., Drogenkunde, W. de Gruyter, 8th ed., 848-851, 1975
18. Nater J.P., De Groot A.C., Unwanted effects of cosmetics and drugs used in dermatology, Excerpta Medica, 314,320, 1983
19. Ravn H., Brimer L., Structure and Antibacterial Activity of Plantamajoside, a caffeic acid sugar ester from *Plantago major* subsp. *major*, Phytochemistry, *27*, 11, 3433-3437,1988
19. Samuelsen A.B. et al., Isolation and Partial Characterisation of Biologically Active Polysaccharides from *Plantago major* L., Phyto therapy Research, *9*, 211-218, 1995
20. DAB 10
21. OAB, '83
22. Ph. Helv. VII
23. BHP '83

Pterocarpus santalinus

Botanical name[1]	*Pterocarpus santalinus* L.
Botanical synonyms	-
Botanical family	Fabaceae
Common names	Red sandalwood (English)
	Rood Sandelhoutboom (Dutch)
	Santal rouge (French)
	Rotes Sandelholz (German)
	Sandalo (Italian)
	Rodt sandeltre (Norwegian)
	Sándalo (Spanish)
EU INCI name[2]	*Pterocarpus santalinus*
CTFA INCI name[3]	Red sandalwood (*Pterocarpus santalinus*) extract

CAS number	84650-41-9
EINECS number	283-511-3
Parts used	Heartwood

Important constituents including active principles[9, 10, 12]

- Essential oil:
  (Sesquiterpenes: α- and β-santalol, cedrol (up to 50%)[9]., pterocarpol, isopterocarpol, pterocarptriol, cryptomeridiol, isopterocarpolone, pterocarpdiolone, α-, β- and γ-eudesmol)
- Triterpenes (acetyl oleanolic acid, acetyl oleanolic aldehyde, erythrodiol, lupendiol)
- Red pigments[14]: santalin A and B, desoxysantalin, pterocarpin, homopterocarpin
- Yellow pigments[15]: santalin Y and AC
- Flavones
- Coumarins
- Tannins
- Phenol acids (chlorogenic, gentisic, caffeic, sinapic, coumaric, ferulic, resorcylic, p-hydroxybenzoic, phloretic, vanillic)
- Phytosterols
- Stilbene derivatives (stilbene, pterostilbene)

Preparation	-
Manufacturing process	-
Examples of specifications	-

Intended cosmetic effects and used concentration in cosmetic products

Astringent, cooling, tonic, dyeing agent, flavour

In tooth powders and mouthwashes as dyeing agent

Other possible effects   Anti-inflammatory, anti-allergic[11], skin diseases (traditional use)[14]

Main toxicological data   No data

Databases used   CA Search 1972-96, Medline 1966-96, Embase 1974-96, Reg. Tox. Eff. Chem. Sub.,Excerpta Medica 1980-96, Life Sciences, Cosmet, Biosis Previews, Cancerlit 1983-96, Toxline, Int. Pharm. Abs.

Keywords   *Pterocarpus santalinus*

Evaluation and remarks   **Cat. B**

General references

1. Index Kewensis, Clarendon Press
2. European Commission Decision 96/335/EC of 8 May 1996, Official Journal of the European Community No. L132 of 1 June 1996
3. International Cosmetic Ingredient Dictionary 6th ed., CTFA, *1*, 1995
4. Council of Europe, Flavouring substances and natural sources of flavourings 3rd ed., Maisonneuve, (379, N2), 1981
5. Grieve M., A modern herbal, Barnes & Noble Books, *2*, 717, 1996
6. Merck Index 12th ed., Merck & Co. Inc., 1996
7. Monograph Santali lignum rubrum, Bundesanzeiger, n.193 (Oct. 15, through Le monografie tedesche, Studio Edizioni, *4*, 1996
8. Proserpio G., Martelli A., Patri G.F., Elementi di fitocosmesi, Sepem, *2*, 1982
9. Van Hellemont J., Compendium de Phytotherapie, APB, 324, 1986
10. Wichtl M., Teedrogen, WVG, 422-423, 1989

Specific references

11. Gupta P.P., Srimal R.C., Tandon J.S., Int. J. Pharmacogn., *31*, n. 1, 1993
12. Hoppe H.A., Drogenkunde, W. de Gruyter, 8th ed., 886-887, 1975
13. Nagaraju N., Prasad M. et al., Blood sugar lowering effect of Pterocarpus santalinus, Int. J. Pharmacognosy, *29*, 141-144, 1991
14. Kambadoor N., Gurudutt and Tiruvenkata R., Seshadri, Phytochemistry, 1974. Vol. 13 pp. 2845 to 2847
15. Junei Kinjo, Hadzuki Uemura and Toshihiro Nohara, Tetrahedron Letters, Vol. 36, No. 31, pp. 5 599-5 602, 1995
16. Ph. B. IV

Rosa aff. rubiginosa

Botanical name[1]	*Rosa* aff. *rubiginosa* L. (sometimes called *Rosa moschata* Herm.)
Botanical synonyms	-
Botanical family	Rosaceae
Common names	Musk Rose (English)
	Myskiruusu (Finnish)
	Rosier musqué (French)
	Moskusrose (German)
	Rosa moscata (Italian)
	Rosa moscada (Spanish)
EU INCI name[2]	*Rosa moschata*
CTFA INCI name[3]	Musk rose (*Rosa moschata*) oil
	Musk rose (*Rosa moschata*) seed oil

CAS number	-
EINECS number	-
Parts used	Seeds

Important constituents including active principles[7]
- Triglycerides containing polyunsaturated fatty acids (oleic 10-20%, cis-linoleic 41-50% and α-linolenic 26-37% acids) and saturated fatty acids (palmitic and stearic acids)
- Vitamin E
- β-Carotene
- Unsaponifiables ($\leq 2.5\%$) (β-sitosterol)

Preparation	Oil
Manufacturing process	Cold pression or solvent extraction and purification
Examples of specifications[7]	Relative density at 20°: 0.924-0.927
	Refractive index at 25°: 1.478-1.482
	Saponification number: 185-195
	Unsaponifiable: not more 2.5%

Intended cosmetic effects and used concentration in cosmetic products
Moisturising, emollient, anti-ageing
Up to 6% in emulsions for fine wrinkle attenuation

Other possible effects	Anti-inflammatory, treatment of skin ulcers[11]
Main toxicological data[7, 6]	Acute oral toxicity: no toxic effects
	Acute dermal toxicity, on rats: no toxic effects

Primary skin irritation: non-irritant
Acute eye irritation: non-irritant
Phototoxicity: no phototoxic effects at skin level
Mutagenicity (test Salmonella typhimurium): no mutagenic effects
Sensitisation: no sensitisation
Photohemolisis: free radical species from the Rosa mosqueta oil lipoperoxidation are postulated to be responsible of the photohemolytic effect obtained[6].

Databases used   CA Search 1967-97, Medline 1966-97, Embase 1974-97, Ref. Tox. Eff. Chem. Sub., Biosis, Toxline, Kosmet, IPA 1970-1997, SCI 1990-1997, Biological Abstract 1992-1997.

Keywords   *Rosa mosqueta, moschata*

Evaluation and remarks   **Cat. A (oil)**

No sign of any toxicity

General references
1. Index Kewensis, Clarendon Press
2. European Commission Decision 96/335/EC of 8 May 1996, Official Journal of the European Community No. L132 of 1 June 1996
3. International Cosmetic Ingredient Dictionary 6th ed., CTFA, 1995
4. Grieve M., A modern herbal, Barnes & Noble Books, 686, 1996
5. Martindale 31st ed., The Royal Pharmaceutical Society, 1996

Specific references
6. Barros S. et al., Photobiological study of Rosa mosqueta oil (Rosa aff. rubiginosa L.), Acta Farm. Bonaerense, *7*, 3-8, 1988
7. ITALCHILE S.r.l. Technical documentation
8. MacDiarmid B.N., Properties and activity of triclopyr on some New Zealand brushweeds, Proc. N. Z. Weed Post Control Conf., *30*, 66-70, 1977
9. Malec L.S. et al., Seeds of Rosa rubiginosa L. Chemical Composition of Seed Oil and Residual Seed Meal, Anales de la Real Academia de Farmacia, *81*, 6, 445-450, 1993
10. Marchini F.B. et al., Effect of Rosa rubiginosa Oil on the Healing of open wound, Revista Paulista de Medicina, *106*, 6, 356, 1988
11. Moreno-Giménez J.C. et al., Tratamiento de las ulceras cutaneas con aceite de rosa de mosqueta, Med. Cutan. Ibero. Lat. Am., *18*, 1, 63-66, 1990
12. Pietta P., Il ruolo degli acidi grassi poliinsaturi e le proprietà della Rosa mosqueta, Erboristeria Domani, *7-8*, 50, 1997
13. Thielemann A.M. et al., Determination of the efficacy of a cream containing Rosa mosqueta oil for wrinkle attenuation, Anales de la Real Academia de Farmacia, *59*, 2, 211-218,1993
14. Villadares J. et al., Cream with oil from mosqueta (Rosa aff. rubiginosa L.) Part 2. study of physicochemical properties, stability, cosmetic efficiency and clinical systematic apllicatio, Anales de la Real Academia de Farmacia, *52*, 3, 597-612, 1986

Rosa centifolia

Botanical name[1]	*Rosa centifolia* L.
Botanical synonyms	-
Botanical family	Rosaceae
Common names	Pale rose (English)
	Centifolia roos (Dutch)
	Kartanoruusu (Finnish)
	Rose pale (French)
	Zentifolien rose (German)
	Rosa pallida (Italian)
	Centifolierose (Norwegian)
	Rosa centifolia (Spanish)
	Centifoliaros (Swedish)
EU INCI name[2]	*Rosa centifolia*
CTFA INCI names[3]	Cabbage rose (*Rosa centifolia*) oil
	Cabbage rose (*Rosa centifolia*) water
	Cabbage rose (*Rosa centifolia*) extract

CAS number	84604-12-6
EINECS number	283-289-8
Parts used	Fresh petals

Important constituents including active principles[9, 15]

- Essential oil (up to 0.04%)[4]:
  (Liquid fraction 75-85%:
  Phenylethylalcohol
  Monoterpenes: α- and β-pinene, myrcene, geraniol, citronellol, nerol and their acetates, linalool, menthol, citral, carvone, rosafurane, neroloxide, cis- and trans- rose oxide
  Sesquiterpenes: farnesol
  Phenol acids and their esters: eugenol, eugenol acetate
  Aldehydes: acetic, benzoic, nonyl aldehydes
  Solid fraction 20-25%:
  Stearoptenes: aliphatic saturated hydrocarbons C_{14}-C_{23} and unsaturated hydrocarbons)
- Flavonoids (anthocyanes)
- Tannins 10-24%[16] (catechic and gallic acids)
- Amino acids
- Mucilages

Preparation

1) Essential oil
2) Distilled water
3) Hydroglycolic extract

Manufacturing process

1) Steam distillation of fresh petals or purification with absolute alcohol of the concrete obtained by extraction with hexane
2) Separation of the aqueous phase after removal of the essential oil
3) Percolation with propylene glycol 50% to final E/D ratio 5:1

Examples of specifications

1) (rose absolute french)[9]:
Specific gravity at 15°C: 0.981 to 0.993
Specific optical rotation: +10° 41' to +13° 10'
Refractive index at 20°C: 1.5096 to 1.5122
Acid number: 3.4 to 7.56
Ester number: 17.5 to 26.6

2)[19] pH: 5.5 to 6.5
Relative density at 20°: 1.038 to 1.042
Refractive index at 20°: 1.388 to 1.392
Dry residue: 0.40 to 1.00%

Intended cosmetic effects and used concentration in cosmetic products

Soothing, astringent, flavour, fragrance

(essential oils)
Up to 0.2%

(glycolic extracts)
Up to 7% in skin care cosmetic products, soaps and detergents for sensitive skin and mucosae, eye contour.

(distilled water)
Up to 20% in lotions and solutions for the treament of eye contour and face with mild astringent and purifying effect.

Other possible effects

Antiseptic, anti-inflammatory[12], anti-microbial

Main toxicological data[16]

(rose absolute french)
LD_{50} oral in rats: > 5000 mg/kg
LD_{50} dermal in rabbits: > 800 mg/kg
Irritation: applied undiluted to the backs of hairless mice and swine it was not irritating. Applied full strength to intact or abraded rabbit skin for 24-hour under occlusion, it was moderately irritating.
Tested at 2% in petrolatum it produced no irritation after 48-hour closed-patch test on human subjects
Sensitisation: A maximisation test was carried out on 25 volunteers. The material was tested at a concentration of 2% in petrolatum and produced no sensitisation reactions.
Phototoxicity: No phototoxic effects were reported for undiluted absolute in hairless mice and swine.

Databases used

CA Search 1967-96, Medline 1966-96, Embase 1974-96, Ref. Tox. Eff. Chem. Sub., Excerpta Medica 1980, Life Sciences, Cosmet, Biosis, Previews, Cancerlit 1983, Toxline, Int. Pharm. Abstracts

Keywords	Rosa centifolia
Evaluation and remarks	**Cat. A**
General references	

1. Index Kewensis, Clarendon Press
2. European Commission Decision 96/335/EC of 8 May 1996, Official Journal of the European Community No. L132 of 1 June 1996
3. International Cosmetic Ingredient Dictionary 6th ed., CTFA, 1995
4. Benigni R., Capra C., Cattorini P.E., Piante Medicinali chimica farmacologia e terapia, Inverni & Della Beffa, *2*, 1360-1362, 1964
5. Council of Europe, Flavouring substances and natural sources of flavourings, 3rd ed Maisonneuve, (404 N2), 1981
6. Flavouring Extract Manufacturers Association (Fema), Survey of flavouring ingredients usage levels, (No.2988), Food Technology, 192 (294), *2*, 1965
7. Fenaroli G., Sostanze Aromatiche Naturali, Hoepli ed., 865-875, 1963
8. Grieve M., A modern herbal, Barnes & Noble Books, *2*, 684-685,689, 1996
9. Guenther E., the essential oils, D. Van Nostrand, *5*, 39-42, 1952
10. Leung A.Y., Foster S., Encyclopedia of common natural ingredients, Wiley & Son Publ., 441-443, 1996
11. Martindale 31st ed., The Royal Pharmaceutical Society, 1996
12. Monograph Rosa flos, Bundesanzeiger, n. 169 (Sept 1, 1990) through Le monografie tedesche, Studio Edizioni, *4*, 1996
13. Paris R.R., Moyse H., Matière Médicale 2nd ed., Masson, *2*, 420,1981
14. Proserpio G., Martelli A., Patri G.F., Elementi di fitocosmesi, Sepem, *2*, 1982
15. Van Hellemont J., Compendium de Phytotherapie, APB, *347*, 1986

Specific references

16. Opdyke D., Food and Cosmetics Toxicology, *12*, 911, 1974
17. Hagars, Handbuch der Pharmazeutischen Praxis, Springer Verlag, 162-1979
18. Hoppe H.A., Drogenkunde, W. de Gruyter, 8th ed., *939*, 1975
19. Indena Product specification, 1996
20. Kreis P. and Mosandl A., Chiral compounds of essential oils: part XII. Authenticity control of rose oils, using enantioselective multidimensional gas chromatography. Flavour and Fragrance Journal, *7*, 199-203,1992
21. Maleev A.T., Todorov S. et al, On the mechanism of the smooth-muscle action of rosanol, Acta Physiologica et Pharmacologica Bulgarica, *13*, 3-1987
22. Wollenweber E., Doerr M., Armbruster S., Flavonoid aglycones as glandular products in Rosa centifolia cv. muscosa and in the Rubus phoenicolasius, Zeitschrift fur Naturforschung Section C Biosciences, 956-958, 1993

Botanical name[1]	*Salix alba* L. and *Salix purpurea* L are the main species used
Botanical synonyms[2] **for *Salix alba***	*Salix vitellina* L.
for *Salix purpurea*	*Salix helix* L.
Other botanical species used	*Salix daphnoides* Vill.
	Salix viminalis L.
	Salix caprea L.
	Salix nigricans Sm.
	Salix fragilis L.
	Salix pentandra L.
Botanical family	Salicaceae

Common names for *Salix alba*

White willow	(English)
Witte Wilg	(Dutch)
Valkopaju	(Finnish)
Saule blanc	(French)
Weiss Weide	(German)
Salice bianco	(Italian)
Hvitpil	(Norwegian)
Sauce blanco	(Spanish)
Vitpil	(Swedish)

for *Salix purpurea*

Red willow	(English)
Bittere Wilg	(Dutch)
Punapaju	(Finnish)
Saule rouge	(French)
Purpur Weide	(German)
Salice rosso	(Italian)
Rødpil	(Norwegian)
Sauce colorado	(Spanish)
Rödvide	(Swedish)

EU INCI name[3]	*Salix alba*
CTFA INCI name[4]	Willow (*Salix alba*) bark extract
	Willow (*Salix alba*) flower extract
	Willow (*Salix alba*) leaf extract
CAS number	84082-82-6 (*Salix alba*)
	84604-23-9 (*Salix purpurea*)

EINECS number 282-029-0 (*Salix alba*)
283-301-1 (*Salix purpurea*)

Parts used Barks and flowers, leaves (sometimes)

Important constituents including active principles[11, 12]

- Phenol glycosides (1,5-11%) (salicin 0,5-10,2%[8], salicortin, tremulacin, populin, fragilin, triandrin, syringin, vimalin, picein, grandidentatin, 3- and 4-acetylsalicortin, salireposide)
- Phenol acids (salicylic, vanillic, syringic, p-hydroxybenzoic, p-coumaric, caffeic and ferulic acid)
- Aldehydes (salidroside, vanillin, syringic aldehyde)
- Alcohols (saligenin)
- Flavonoids (isoquercitrin, naringin, isosalipurposide, quercetin and isorhamnetin glucosides)[21]
- Biflavones[20]
- Catechic tannins 8-20%[11, 12]
- Oligo and polysaccharides[22, 23]: (contain mainly galactan and arabinan, pectins)

Preparation[5] 1) Fluid extract E/D = 1:1
2) Dry aqueous extract E/D = 1:10

Manufacturing process 1) Extraction with alcohol 30% and concentration under vacuum to final E/D ratio 1:1
2) Extraction with water and concentration under vacuum to dryness

Examples of specifications

Intended cosmetic effects and used concentration in cosmetic products
Moisturising, keratolitic, purifying
Up to 20% in products for hardened skin and corns in emulsions and mask for face and body
Up to 0.5% as preservative

Other possible effects Astringent, analgesic, anti-inflammatory, granulation promoting agent[11], antimicrobial

Main toxicological data[17] (*S. alba*, stem bark extract):
LD_{50} i.p. in mice: 375 mg/kg.(RTECS)

(Salicylates and salicin)[8, 19]
Hypersensitivity reactions to salicylates. Systemic poisoning has occured from the application of salicylates to large areas of skin

Databases used CA Search 1967-96, Medline 1966-96, Embase 1974-96, Reg. Tox. Eff. Chem. Sub.,Excerpta Medica 1980-96, Life Science, Cosmet, Biosis Previews, Cancerlit 1983-96, Toxline, Int. Pharm. Abstracts

Keywords *Salix alba*

Evaluation and remarks **Cat. A (if salicylate and salicylate generators free)**

General references

1. Index Kewensis, Clarendon Press
2. Penso G., Index Plantarum Medicinalium Totius Mundi Eorumque Synonymorum, OEMF, 1983
3. European Commission Decision 96/335/EC of 8 May 1996, Official Journal of the European Community No. L132 of 1 June 1996
4. International Cosmetic Ingredient Dictionary 6th ed., CTFA, 2, 1995
5. Benigni R., Capra C., Cattorini P.E., Piante Medicinali chimica farmacologia e terapia, Inverni & Della Beffa, 2, 1 397-1 401, 1964
6. Grieve M., A modern herbal, Barnes & Noble Books, 2, 847, 1996
7. Martindale 31st ed., The Royal Pharmaceutical Society, 1996
8. Monograph Salix cortex, Bundesanzeiger, No. 228 (Dec 05, 1984) through Le monografie tedesche, Studio Edizioni, 2, 1994
9. Newall C., Anderson L., Phillipson J.D., Herbal Medicines: a guide for health care professionals, The Pharmaceutical Press, 268-269, 1996
10. Paris R.R., Moyse H., Matière Médicale 2nd ed., Masson, 2, 89-90, 1981
11. Van Hellemont J., Compendium de Phytotherapie, APB, 357-359, 1986
12. Wichtl M., Teedrogen, WVG, 516-518, 1989

Specific references

13. FAO/WHO Joint Expert Committee in Food additives, 1961
14. Goncalo S., Sousa J., Monero A., Leitao A., Occupational dermatitis from Salix viminalis, Contact Dermatitis, 14, 188-189, 1986
15. Hagers, Handbuch der Pharmazeutischen Praxis, Springer-Verlag,
16. Hoppe H. A., Drogenkunde 8th ed., W. de Gruyter, 955-957, 1975
17. Nater J.P., De Groot A. C., Unwanted Effects of cosmetics and drugs used in Dermatology, Excerpta Medica, 316, 320, 1983
18. Shimizu Matsuzawa T., et al., Studies on bathing agents: 1. Anti-inflammatory effect of bathing agents used for skin disease, Shoyakugaku Zasshi, 47, 1-4, 1993
19. Recommendations concerning undesirable active principles, 3.1, 28th meeting Committee of Experts on Cosmetic Products, Rome, 3-7 November 1997, Council of Europe
20. Imdam u., Khan and W. H. Ansari, Biflavonoid from the Family Salicaceae, j. Indian Chem. Soc., Vol. LXII, September 1985
21. Christian Karl., et al., Flavonoide aus Salix alba. Die Struktur des terniflorius und eines weiteren acylflavonoides, Phytochemistry, 1976. Vol. 15, pp. 1084-1085

22. Toman R., et. Al., Polysaccharides from the bark of the white willow (Salix alba L.): Structure of a galactan, Carbohydrate Research, 25 (1972), 371-378
23. Karácsonyi S, et. al., Polysaccharides from the bark of the bark of the white willow (Salix alba L.): Structure of an arabinan, Carbohydrate Research, 44 (1975) 285-290
24. BPC '34
25. Br. Herb. Ph. 1990
26. DAB 10

Sambucus nigra

Botanical name[1]	*Sambucus nigra* L.
Botanical synonyms[2]	*Sambucus vulgaris* Neck.
Botanical family	Caprifoliaceae

Common names

Black Elder	(English)
Vlier	(Dutch)
Sureau noir	(French)
Schwarzer Holunder	(German)
Sambuco nero	(Italian)
Svarthyll	(Norwegian)
Saúco	(Spanish)
Fläder	(Swedish)

EU INCI name[3]   *Sambuscus nigra*

CTFA INCI name[4]

Sambucus nigra
Sambucus nigra extract
Sambucus nigra berry extract
Sambucus nigra oil
Sambucus nigra water

CAS number	84603-58-7 (extract)
	68916-55-2 (oil)
EINECS number	2832594
Parts used	Flowers and fruits

Important constituents including active principles[12., 16.]

Flowers:

– Essential oil (up to 0.3%)[12., 29.]
(Fatty acids: palmitic, linoleic and linolenic acids
Hydrocarbons: C_{19}, C_{21}, C_{23} and C_{25} alkanes
Terpenes)

– Triterpenes (up to 2%)[15.] (α- and β-amyrin, lupeol, cycloartenol, 2,4-methylenecycloartenol, cycloeucalenol, ursolic, 30-β-hydrox-yursolic acid, oleanolic acids) in free form or esterfied form or as glycosides

– Phytosterols (up to 0.1%)[15.] (cholesterol, campesterol, stigmasterol and β-sitosterol) in free form or as glycosides

– Flavonoids (up to 2%)[15.] (rutin, isoquercitrin, astragalin, quercetin, kaempferol, isorhamnetin-3-O-rutinoside and isorhamnetin-3-O-glucoside)

– Phenol acids (chlorogenic (3%)[20], caffeic, ferulic and p-coumaric acids)
– Tannins
– Pectins
– Sugars
– Amines (ethylamine, isobutylamine)
– Choline
– Vitamin C

Fruits:
– Anthocyanosides (sambucin (0.2-1%)[20, 25], sambucyanin, cyanin, chrysanthemin, keracyanin, sambunigrin)
– Flavonoids (rutin and isoquercitrin)
– Triterpenes (α-amyrin, betulin, α-amyrone, ursolic acid)
– Phenolic acid (shikimic and chlorogenic acids)
– Amino acids (tyrosine)
– Organic acids (malic, malonic, lactic, oxalic, citric, tartaric, quinic, valerianic)
– Mineral salts
– Vitamins (B group, C, P, H, folic acid, PP)
– β-carotene
– Lectins[24]
– Tannins (up to 3%)[19]
– Sugars (7.5%)[20] (levulose)
– Pectin (3%)[11]

Preparation

1) Sambucus extract[6]
2) Hydroalcoholic fluid extract ratio E/D 1:1[16]
3) Distilled water[12]

Manufacturing process

1) Extraction from flowers or sap fruits with propylene glycol, 1,3-butylene glycol ortheir aqueous solutions
2) Extraction from flowers with alcohol 25% and concentration under vacuum to final E/D ratio 1:1
3) Water collected from steam distillate of flowers

Examples of specifications

1) Heavy metals: not more than 20 ppm
Arsenic: not more than 2 ppm

Intended cosmetic effects and used concentration in cosmetic products

Mild tonic, astringent, refreshing, soothing, protective, moisturising, dyeing agent (fruits)

(distilled water)

In lotions for eye contour and products for delicate skin (as a vehicle). For clearing the complexion of freckles and sunburns (traditional use)

(extract)

In products for chapped hands, skin fresheners, pre-sun products, gargles and mouthwashes

Other possible effects

Diaphoretic, diuretic, granulation-promoting agent, anti-inflammatory, venous astringent, antihaemorrhoidal (traditional use)

Main toxicological data	(berries) Cause nausea and vomiting

(fresh flowers)
Are irritant to the skin

(rutin and quercetin)
LD_{50} oral in mice: 4000 mg/kg [24.]
LD_{50} i.v. in mice: 950 mg/kg [24.]
carcinogenicity test: rutin is suggested to be biotransformed to quercetin, which is supposed to be mutagenic and carcinogenic.
Quercetin has been tested for carcinogenicity in a number of animal species and through several administration routes. An increased incidence of tumours has been observed in only one experiment in rats fed quercetin, whereas several other experiments using the same or higher doses did not provide any evidence of carcinogenic effects.
Rutin (the 3-rhamnoglucoside of quercetin) was tested in rats and hamsters with no evidence of carcinogenicity.

The *in vitro* pattern of genotoxicity of quercetin for different genetic endpoints is subject to a variety of factors such as pH, antioxidants, metabolism and nitrosation, whose role in each test system remains unclear, but evidence of *in vivo* mutagenicity of quercetin is still lacking.
Quercetin and other flavonoids have also been reported to have a number of positive effects including eicosanoid biosynthesis modification, protection of low-density lipoproteins from oxidation, prevention of platelet aggregation and promotion of relation of cardiovascular smooth muscle.[29.]

Both berries and flowers have long been used, apparently safely, after they have been cooked.[24.]

Databases used

CA Search 1967-96, Medline 1966-96, Embase 1974-96, Ref. Tox. Eff. Chem. Sub., Toxline, Napralert, Cosmet

Keywords

Sambucus nigra

Evaluation and remarks

Cat B

General references

1. Index Kewensis, Clarendon Press
2. Penso G., Index Plantarum Medicinalium Totius Mundi Eorumque Synonymorum, OEMF, 1983
3. European Commission Decision 96/335/EC of 8 May 1996, Official Journal of the European Community No. L132 of 1 June 1996
4. International Cosmetic Ingredient Dictionary 6th ed., CTFA, *1*, 1995
5. Benigni R., Capra C., Cattorini P.E., Piante Medicinali chimica farmacologia e terapia, Inverni & Della Beffa, *2*, 1421-1424, 1964
6. Comprehensive Licensing Standards of Cosmetics by Category, Yakuji Nippo Ltd., *1*, 266, 1986

145

7. Council of Europe, Flavouring substances and natural sources of flavourings 3rd ed., Maisonneuve, (417, N2), 1981
8. Flavouring Extract Manufacturers Association (Fema), Survey of flavouring ingredients usage levels, (No. 2 406), Food Technology, 170 (272), 1965
9. Fenaroli G., Le sostanze aromatiche, Hoepli ed., 894-895, 1963
10. Grieve M., A modern herbal, Barnes & Noble Books, 265-276, 1996
11. Japanese Cosmetic Ingredient Codex, Yakuji Nippo, Ltd, 754, 1993
12. Leung A.Y., Foster S., Encyclopedia of common natural ingredients Wiley & Son Publ., 220-222, 1996
13. Martindale 31st ed., The Royal Pharmaceutical Society, 1996
14. Merck Index 12th ed., Merck & Co. Inc., 1996
15. Monograph Sambuci flos, Bundesanzeiger, No. 50 (Mar 13, 1986) trough Le monografie tedesche, Studio Edizioni, *4*, 1996
16. Newall C., Anderson L., Phillipson J.D., Herbal Medicines a guide for health care professionals, The Pharmaceutical Press, 104-105, 1996
17. Paris R.R., Moyse H., Matière Médicale, Masson ed., *3*, 384-385, 1981
18. Proserpio G., Martelli A., Patri G.F., Elementi di fitocosmesi, Sepem, *2*, 1982
19. Van Hellemont J., Compendium de Phytotherapie, APB, 361-363, 1986
20. Wichtl M., Teedrogen, WVG, 237-238, 1989

Specific references

21. Beckstrom-Sternberg S.M., Duke J.A., "The Phytochemical Database"
22. Bisset N.G., Herbal drugs and Phytopharmaceuticals, Medpharm Scientific Publ., 1994
23. CE Data sheets, Nov. 1996
24. Hansen K.B., Hansen S.H., High-performance liquid chromatographic separation of anthocyanins of *Sambucus nigra* L., Journal of Chromatography, 262, 385-392, 1983
25. Juhos T., Wladimir E., Kristof I., Pal V., Synergistic sunscreen comprising *Sambucus nigra* extract, Austrian AT 393,451, 25 Oct 1991
26. Mach L., et al., Purification and partial characterization of a novel lectin from elder (*Sambucus nigra* L.) fruit, Biochem. J., 278, 667-671, 1991
27. Nater J.P., De Groot A.C., Unwanted effects of cosmetics and drugs used in dermatology, Excerpta Medica, 314,320, 1983
28. Toulemonde B., Hubert M.J. Richard, Volatile Constituents of Dry Elder (*Sambucus nigra* L.) Flowers, J. Agric. Food Chem., *31*, 365-370, 1983
29. Recommendations concerning undesirable active principles, 3.16, 28th meeting Committee of Experts on Cosmetic Products, Rome, 3-7 November 1997, Council of Europe.

30. Ph. Fr. X
31. Ph. Helv VII, '94
32. DAC '86
33. OAB '83
34. Ph Ned 5, 6
35. Ph B II, IV
36. BHP, '90
37. Ph Bg VII

Saponaria officinalis

Botanical name[1]	*Saponaria officinalis* L.
Botanical synonyms[1]	*Saponaria vulgaris* Pall.
Botanical family	Caryophyllaceae
Common names	Soapwort (English)
	Zeepkruid (Dutch)
	Suopayrtti (Finnish)
	Savonnière (French)
	Seifenkraut (German)
	Saponaria (Italian)
	Såpeurt (Norwegian)
	Saponella (Spanish)
	Såpnejlika (Swedish)
EU INCI name[3]	*Saponaria officinalis*
CTFA INCI name[4]	*Saponaria officinalis* extract

CAS number	84775-97-3
EINECS number	283-921-2
Parts used	Roots, leaves (sometimes)

Important constituents including active principles[5, 14, 15]
- Essential oil
- Flavonoids (saponarine in leaves)
- Triterpene saponins (saponaroside) and genins (quillaic acid, gipsogenin) (up to 5%)[14]
- Proteins (saporin)[16]
- Organic acids (glycolic and glyceric acids)
- Sugars
- Mucilages (galactomannans)
- Calcium oxlate

Preparation
1) Saponaria extract[6]
2) Fluid extact E/D = 1:1[5]

Manufacturing process
1) Extraction of leaves with propylene glycol, 1,3-butylene glycol or their mixture
2) Extraction of roots with alcohol 20% and concentration to final ratio E/D 1:1

Examples of specifications
1)[6] Heavy metals: not more than 20 ppm
   Arsenic: not more than 2 ppm

Intended cosmetic effects and used concentration in cosmetic products

Foaming, surfactant, emulsifying, soothing, purifying, anti-itching
Up to 10% in products for oily and impure skin, emulsions and gels for cellulitis, detergents for sensitive skin and scalp, cleaning and freshening lotion

Other possible effects

Anti-inflammatory, anti-oedema, antiseborroic, antiviral[18.]

Main toxicological data

LD_{50} oral in rats: 3000 mg/kg[16.]
Subchronic toxicity: LDL0 subcutaneous in mice: 900 mg/kg[16.]
LDL_0 i.v. in mice: 1000 mg/kg[16.]
LDL_0 i.v. in cats: 46 mg/kg[16.]
LDL_0 i.v. in rabbits: 40 mg/kg[16.]
TDL_0 i.p. in rats: 350 mg/kg[30.]

(saponins)[24.]:
Acute eye irritation: conjunctivitis and damage of the cornea
Skin irritation: irritant to mucous membranes
Mixture of hydropropylenglycol or hydrobutylenglycol extract containing 5% of 1)[17.]:
Primary skin irritation on rabbits: non-irritant
Acute eye irritation on rabbits: non-irritant
According to the Commission E monograph, the use of Saponaria officinalis (aerial parts) is not recommended because of lack of documentation.[11.]

Databases used

CA Search 1967-95, Medline 1966-95, Embase 1974-95, Reg. Tox. Eff. Chem. Sub, Napralert, Toxline, Cosmet

Keywords

Saponaria officinalis

Evaluation and remarks

Cat. B

General references

1. Index Kewensis, Clarendon Press
2. Penso G., Index Plantarum Medicinalium Totius Mundi Eorumque Synonymorum, OEMF, 1983
3. Inventario Europeo degli Ingredienti Cosmetici, Unipro, 2, 1995
4. International Cosmetic Ingredient Dictionary 6th ed., CTFA, 2, 1995
5. Benigni R., Capra C., Cattorini P.E., Piante Medicinali chimica farmacologia e terapia, Inverni & Della Beffa, 2, 1432-1436, 1964
6. Comprehensive Licensing Standards of Cosmetics by Category, Yakuji Nippo Ltd., 1, 266, 1986
7. Council of Europe, Flavouring substances and natural sources of flavourings 3rd ed., Maisonneuve,(422,N3), 1981
8. Grieve M., A modern herbal, Barnes & Noble Books, 2, 748, 1996
9. Japanese Cosmetic Ingredients Codex, Yukuji Nippo, LTD., 754-755, 1993
10. Merck Index 12th ed., Merck & Co. Inc., 1996

11. Monograph Saponariae herba - Saponariae rubrae radix, Bundesanzeiger, No. 80 (Apr., 27, 1989) through Le monografie tedesche, Studio Edizioni, *3*, 1995

12. Paris R.R., Moyse H., Matière Médicale 2nd ed., Masson, *2*, 315, 1981

13. Proserpio G., Martelli A., Patri G.F., Elementi di fitocosmesi, Sepem, *2*, 696,1982

14. Van Hellemont J., Compendium de Phytotherapie, APB, 366-368, 1986

15. Wichtl M., Teedrogen, WVG, 443-444, 1989

Specific references

16. Abbernalden Handbuch der Biologischen Arzneimittel

17. AEL P.A. de Smet, Adverse Effects of Herbal Drugs, Springer Verlag Heidelberg, *2*, 1992

18. Back P., The Illustrated Herbal, Hamlyn Publ., 1987

19. Barthelemy I., Martineau D. et al., The Expression of Saponin, a Ribosome-inactivating Protein from the Saponaria officinalis, in Escherichia coli, The Journal of Biological Chemistry, 268, 9, 6 541-6 548, 1993

20. Biolab unpublished report (Phytelene complexe peaux grasses)

21. Bisset NG (Ed), Herbal drugs and Phytopharmaceuticals: Medpharm Scientific Publi., CRC Press, 1994

22. Bremness L., The complete book of herbs, Colour Library Books Dorling Kindersley Ltd.

23. Bunney S., The Illustrated Book of Herbs, Octopus, 1984

24. FYC Fyto therapeutisch Compendium, 2nd edition, BohmStafleu-van Logchem, Houten/Zaventem, 1988

25. KHF Der kosmos-Heilpflanzenfuhrer, Europaische Heil-und Giftpflanzen, Franckh-Kosmos, 5 e Aufl., 1991

26. Pinkhof, van der Wielen, Pharmacotherapeutisch Vademecum, unieboek BV, Bussum, 1979

27. Potterton D., Culpeper's Colour Herbal, W. Foulsham, 1983

28. Nater J.P., De Groot A.C., Unwanted effects of cosmetics and drugs used in dermatology, Excerpta Medica, 316, 1983

29. Serkedjieva J., Manolova N., Antiviral Activity of Infusion (SHS-174) from Flowers of *Sambucus nigra* L., Aerial parts of Hypericum perforatum L., and Roots of Saponaria officinalis L., against Influenza and Herpes Simplex Viruses, Phytotherapy Research, *4*, 3, 97-100, 1990

30. Texas Reports on Biology

31. Ph. Fr. X

38. Ph B II

33. DAC '86

34. BPC 54

Silybum marianum

Botanical name[1]	*Silybum marianum* (L.) Gaertn.
Botanical synonyms[2]	*Carduus marianus* L. Botanical family Asteraceae
Common names	Milk thistle (English)
	Maria Distel (Dutch)
	Maarianohdake (Finnish)
	Chardon Marie (French)
	Mariendistel (German)
	Cardo mariano (Italian)
	Maritistel ((Norwegian)
	Cardo de María (Spanish)
	Mariatistel (Swedish)
EU INCI names[3]	*Silybum marianum*
CTFA INCI names[4]	Lady's thistle (*Silybum maranium*) extract

CAS number	84604-20-6
EINECS number	283-298-7
Parts used	Fruits

Important constituents including active principles[8, 9, 17]
- Essential oil (0,1%)[10]
- Silymarin (1.5-3%)[17] (flavanolignans) (silybin A and B, 2,3-dehydrosilybin, 2,3-dehydrosilychristin, isosilybin A and B, silydianin, silychristin, isosilychristin, siliermin, silymonin, silandrin, neosiliermin A and B) and flavanolignans oligomers (tri-, tetra- and pentamers) and flavonoids (quercetin[18], taxifolin, dehydrokaempferol)
- Dehydroxyconiferyl alcohol
- Triglycerides (20-30%)[17] (cont. linolenic acid, linoleic, oleic, palmitic, arachic, galacturonic acid)
- Alkaloids
  Saponins
- Protein (26-28%)[9] (albumin, histamine, tyramine)
- Polysaccharides (containing arabinose, rhamnose, xylose, glucose)
- Sesquiterpenes
- Phytosterols (0.6%)[10] (b-sitosterol, stigmasterol, campesterol, cholesterol)
- Sugars
- Vitamins (C, E and K)

Preparation	Purified dry extract (Silymarin)

Manufacturing process Percolation with aceton and purification with hexane

Examples of specifications Silymarin: not less than 65%
Loss on drying: not more than 5%
Sulphated ash: not more than 1%
Heavy metals: not more than 20 ppm
Arsenic: not more than 2 ppm

Intended cosmetic effects and used concentration in cosmetic products
Anti-ageing, skin protectant, purifying, anti-dandruff
Up to 3% in products for impure and oily skin, pre-sun products

Other possible effects Anti-oxidant, anti-inflammatory, free radical scavenger, anti-bacterial[16], protective of cells membrane, antielastase

Main toxicological data[12, 15, 14] A seed extract administered i.m. to mice (1 ml every day for a week) did not show any toxic effect.[11]

(Silymarin)
LD_{50} i.p. in mice: 681 mg/kg (RTECS)
LD_{50} i.p. in rats: 1915 mg/kg
LD_{50} oral in mice: > 20000 mg/kg
  in dogs: > 1000 mg/kg
  in rats: > 5000 mg/kg
Primary skin irritation in rabbits: non-irritant
Acute eye irritation in rabbits: non-irritant
Skin sensibilisation in guinea pigs: non-sensitising
Sub-chronic toxicity in rats: no adverse effect of oral dose of 1000 mg/kg per 15 days. No adverse effect of oral route of 100 mg/kg/day per 16 or 22 weeks
Embryotoxic effects in rats and in rabbits: no evidence

Databases used CA Search 1967-96, Medline 1966-96, Embase 1974-96, Reg. Tox. Eff. Chem. Sub.

Keywords *Silybum marianum*

Evaluation and remarks Cat. A (purified dry extract) Well-known plant, used internally as anti-hepatotoxic, with no toxic effects. The same applies to external use.

General references
1. Index Kewensis, Clarendon Press
2. Penso G., Index Plantarum Medicinalium Totius Mundi Eorumque Synonymorum, OEMF, 1983
3. European Commission Decision 96/335/EC of 8 May 1996, Official Journal of the European Community No. L132 of 1 June 1996
4. International Cosmetic Ingredient Dictionary 6th ed., CTFA, *1*, 1995
5. Grieve M., A modern herbal, Barnes & Noble Books, *2*, 797, 1996
6. Martindale 31st ed., The Royal Pharmaceutical Society, 1996
7. Merck Index 12th ed., Merck & Co. Inc., 1996

8. Monograph Cardui mariae fructus, Bundesanzeiger, No. 50 (March 13, 1986) through Le monografie tedesche, Studio Edizioni, *1*, 1994

9. Leung A.Y., Foster S., Encyclopedia of common natural ingredients, Wiley & Son Publ., 366-368, 1996

10. Van Hellemont J., Compendium de Phytotherapie, APB, 80-81, 1986

11. Wichtl M., Teedrogen, WVG, 331-333, 1989

Specific references

12. Akak Nauk, Azerbidzzhan SSR, *6*, 71-75, 1954

13. Betés C., Benaiges, Estudio de actividad y estabilidad de la silibina, 1st Congres Mediterranéen de Cosmetologie, La Grande Motte, Société Française de Cosmétologie, J.J. Etienne/J.P. Marty, 1996

14. De Vincenzi M., Dessi M.R., Botanical flavouring substances used in foods: proposal of classification Silybum marianum (L.) Gaertn., Fitoterapia, *65*, 1, 54-55, 1994

15. Hahn G., Lehmann H.D., Kurten M., Uebel H. and Vogel G., Zur Pharmakologie und Toxikologie von Silymarin, des antihepatotoxischen Wirkprinzipes aus Silybum marianum L. Gaertn., Arzneim. Forsch., *18*, 6, 698-704, 1968

16. Indena specifications

17. Izzo A.A., Di Carlo G. et al., Biological screening of Italian medicinal plants for antibacterial activity, Phyto ther. Res., 9, 281-286, 1995

18. Morazzoni P., Bombardelli E.- Silybum marianum (Carduus marianus) (review), Fitoterapia LXVI, 1, 3-42, 1995

19. Recommendations concerning undesirable active principles, 3.16, 28th meeting Committee of Experts on Cosmetic Products, Rome, 3-7 November 1997, Council of Europe.

20. FU IX

21. Ph. Fr. X

22. DAB X

Syzygium aromaticum

Botanical name[1]	*Syzygium aromaticum* (L.) Merr. et Perr.
Botanical synonyms[2]	*Eugenia caryophyllus* (Spr.) Bull. et Harr., *Caryophyllus aromaticus* L., *Eugenia aromatica* Baill., *Eugenia caryophyllata*thunb., *Jambosa caryophyllus* Nied., *Myrtus caryophyllus* Spr.)
Botanical family	Myrtaceae
Common names	Clove (English)
	Kruidnagel (Dutch)
	Mausteneilikka (Finnish)
	Giroflier (French)
	Gewürznelkenbaum (German)
	Garofano (Italian)
	Kriddernelliktre (Norwegian)
	Clavo (Spanish)
	Kryddnejlika (Swedish)
EU INCI name[3]	*Eugenia caryophyllus*
CTFA INCI name[4]	Clove (*Eugenia caryophyllus*) extract
	Clove (*Eugenia caryophyllus*) oil
	Clove leaf (*Eugenia caryophyllus*) oil

CAS number	84961-50-2 (extract)
	8000-34-8 (essential oil)
	8015-97-2 (essential oil)
EINECS number	284-638-7
Parts used	Buds, (leaves and stems)

Important constituents including active principles[14, 22, 28]

- Essential oil (up to 20%)[22]:
  Monoterpenes (eugenol 85-95%[22], isoeugenol, methyleugenol, eugenyl acetate up to 3%[19], chavicol)
  Sesquiterpenes (β-caryophyllene 5-12%[20], epoxycaryophyllene, α-ylangene)
  Ketons (eugenone, methylamylketone, methylheptylketone)
  Aldehydes (benzaldehyde, furfural)
  Methyl salicylate
- Flavonoids (quercetin, kaempferol, rhamnetin)[37]
- Tannins (10-12%)[21]
- Phenol acids (gallic and protocatechic acids)
- Phytosterols (β-sitosterol, stigmasterol, campesterol) as glycosides
- Lipids (up to 20%)[20]

– Chromones (eugenin, eugenitin, isoeugenitol, isoeugenitin)
– Triterpene acids (oleanolic and crataegolic acids)[24, 35]
– Vitamins
– Mucilages
– Sugars
– Proteins (about 6%)[20]
– Waxes and resins

Preparation

1) Essential oil
2) Clove extract[7]

Manufacturing process

1) Water or steam distillation of buds[7, 10]
2) Extraction of dried buds with ethanol solution[7]

Examples of specifications

1)[10] Specific gravity at 25°: 1.051
   Specific optical rotation: - 0° 32'
   Refractive index at 20°: 1.5318
   Solubility: complete in 1 vol. alcohol 70%
   Phenols total cont.: 91%
2)[7] Heavy metals: not more than 20 ppm.
   Arsenic: not more than 2 ppm

Intended cosmetic effects and used concentration in cosmetic products

Purifying agent, fragrance

(Essential oil)
Up to 0.25% in soap and detergents, in toothpastes, massage preparations

(Extract)
Up to 5% in mouthwashes and breath fresheners, cosmetic lotions and shampoos, skin care products, cleansing products and preparation for impure skin

Other possible effects

Anti-microbial, anti-fungal[25, 26, 27], anti-histaminic, spasmolytic, analgesic (in dentistry undiluted essential oil), antioxidant[30, 36], tripsin-potentiating activity,[31, 32] in treatment of athlete's foot

Main toxicological data

(Essential oil from buds)[33]
LD_{50}, oral in rats: 372 mg/100 g
LD_{50}, dermal in rabbits: approx. 5000 mg/kg
Clove oil was toxic to mice when applied to the skin in two doses 7 days apart.
Chronic toxicity: daily oral doses of 35 or 70 mg clove oil given for 8 weeks were tolerated by rats. At higher doses there was inactivity leading to weight loss. Death accompanied by severe liver and kidney changes occured after 2-3 weeks on 105 mg/day and rapidly followed one dose of 140 mg.
Skin irritation: (undiluted oil) on hairless mice: not irritating.
Full strength, intact or abraded rabbits skin 24 hours under occlusion: moderately irritating
Human: closed-patch test, 20% petrolatum or ointment:
Primary irritation (erythema) 2 out of 25 subjects.

30 normal subjects (2% concentration): no reactions.

35 subjects with dermatosis (0.2% concentration): no reactions

Human subjects, 5% petrolatum 48 hrs closed-patch test: no reactions

Sensitisation-man: Maximisation (25 volunteers, 5% petrolatum): no reactions. Sensitisation of human skin caused by clove oil was attributed to the presence of eugenol.

Phototoxicity: (undiluted oil), on hairless mice and swine: no effects.

(Methyleugenol)

Carcinogenic in pre-weaned mice, inducing liver tumours.

Mutagenic in several systems[39.]

(Isogenol)[38.]

Up to 0.2%

(quercetin, rutin)

Quercetin has been tested for carcinogenicity in a number of animal species and through several administration routes. An increased incidence of tumours has been observed in only one experiment in rats fed quercetin, whereas several other experiments using the same or higher doses did not provide any evidence of carcinogenic effects.

Rutin (the 3-rhamnoglucoside of quercetin) was tested in rats and hamsters with no evidence of carcinogenicity.

The in vitro pattern of genotoxicity of quercetin for different genetic endpoints is subject to a variety of factors such as pH, antioxidants, metabolism and nitrosation, whose role in each test system remains unclear, but evidence of in vivo mutagenicity of quercetin is still lacking.

Quercetin and other flavonoids have also been reported to have a number of positive effects including eicosanoid biosynthesis modification, protection of low-density lipoproteins from oxidation, prevention of platelet aggregation and promotion of relation of cardiovascular smooth muscle.[40.]

Databases used

CA Search 1967-95, Medline 1966-95, Embase 1974-95, Ref. Tox. Eff. Chem. Sub., Biosis, Toxline, Kosmet

Keywords

Syzygium aromaticum, Clove

Evaluation and remarks

Cat. A (extract)
Essential oil: no final decision

Despite its anaesthetic, anti-inflammatory and bactericidal properties, the essential oil may, when placed in direct contact with live tissues, cause histological lesions, as a result of which some dentists no longer use it. Its external use should be limited, particularly in children. The extract, on the other hand, contains much less essential oil and its use may be considered to be relatively safe.

General references

1. Index Kewensis, Clarendon Press
2. Penso G., Index Plantarum Medicinalium Totius Mundi Eorumque Synonymorum, OEMF, 1983
3. European Commission Decision 96/335/EC of 8 May 1996, Official Journal of the European Community No. L132 of 1 June 1996
4. International Cosmetic Ingredient Dictionary 6th ed., CTFA, 1,1995
5. Benigni R., Capra C., Cattorini P.E., Piante Medicinali chimica farmacologia e terapia, Inverni & Della Beffa, *1*, 633- 636, 1971
6. Comprehensive Licensing Standards of Cosmetics by Category, Yakuji Nippo Ltd., *1*, 40, 1986
7. Comprehensive Licensing Standards of Cosmetics by Category, Yakuji Nippo Ltd., *6*, 92, 1992
8. Council of Europe, Flavouring substances and natural sources of flavourings 3rd ed. Maisonneuve, (188 N2), 1981
9. Flavouring Extract Manufactures Association (Fema), Survey of flavouring ingredients usage levels, (No. 2322,2323, 2324, 2325, 2327, 2328), Food Technology, 167 (269), 1965
10. Fenaroli G., Sostanze Aromatiche Naturali, Hoepli, 576-584, 1963
11. Grieve M., A modern herbal, Barnes & Noble Books, 208, 1996
12. Guenther E., the essential oils, D. Van Nostrand, *4*, 412-422, 1952
13. The Japanese Cosmetic Ingredients Codex, ed. Yakuji Nippo Ltd., 154, 1993
14. Leung A.Y., Foster S, Encyclopedia of Common Natural Ingredients, Wiley & Son Publ., 174-177, 1996
15. Martindale 31st ed., The Royal Pharmaceutical Society, 1996
16. Merck Index 12th ed., Merck & Co. Inc., 1996
17. Monographs Caryophylli flos, Bundesanzeiger , No. 223 (Nov. 30, 1985), through Le monografie tedesche, Studio Edizioni, *4*, 1996
18. Newall C., Anderson L., Phillipson J.D., Herbal Medicines a guide for health care professionals, The Pharmaceutical Press, *79*, 1996
19. Paris R.R., Moyse H., Matière Mèdicale, Masson ed., *2*, 443-446, 1981
20. Proserpio G., Martelli A., Patri G.F., Elementi di fitocosmesi, Sepem, *2*, 681- 682, 1983
21. Van Hellemont J., Compendium de Phytotherapie, APB, 84-86, 1986
22. Wichtl M., Teedrogen, WVG, 193-194, 1989

Specific references

23. Arctander S., Perfume and Flavor Materials of natural origin, 1960
24. Brieskorn C.H., Münzhuber K., Unger G., Crataegolsäure und Steroidglukoside aus Blütenknospen von *Syzygium aromaticum*, Phytochemistry, *14*, 2308-2309, 1975
25. Cai L., Wu C.D., Compounds from *Syzygium aromaticum* Possessing Growth Inhibitory Activity Against Oral Pathogens, J.Nat.Prod., *59*, 987-990, 1996

26. Cai L., Park W., Wu-Yuan C.D., Antimicrobial Compound from *Syzygium aromaticum* (Clove) Inhibit Oral Pathogens, 96th General meet. of the Am. Soc. Microbiol. New Orleans, May 19-23, 265, 1996

27. Deans S.G., Noble R.C. and al., Antimicrobial and Antioxidant Properties of *Syzygium aromaticum* (L.) Merr. & Perry: Impact upon Bacteria, Fungi and Fatty Acid Levels in Aging Mice, Flavour and Fragrance Journal., *10*, 323-328, 1995

28. Gaydou E.M., Randriamiharisoa R.P., Multidimensional Analysis of Gas Chromatographic Data, Application to the Differentiation of Clove Bud and Clove Stem Essential Oils from Madagascar, Perfumer & Flavorist, *12*, 45-51, 1987

29. de Groot A.C., Weyland JW, Nater J.P., Unwanted effects of cosmetics and drugs used in dermatology, 3 ed., Elsevier Science Publishers B.V., 1994

30. Hirahara F., Takai Y., Iwao H., Antioxidative activity of various spices on oils and fats I. Antioxidative activity for storage and heating, through Chem. Abstr. *82*, 2764u, 1975

31. Kato Y., Effects of spice extracts on hydrolases. I On trypsin, through Chem. Abstr. *84*, 149393x, 1976

32. Kato Y., Effects of spice extracts on hydrolases. II Effects of essential oils of clove,thyme, and all spice on trypsin, through Chem. Abstr. 84, 178343m, 1976

33. Opdyke D.L.J., Monographs on Fragrance Raw Materials, Clove Bud oil, Food and Cosmetics Toxicology, *13*, 761-763, 1975

34. Masada Y., Analysis of essential oils by Gas Chromatography and Mass Spectrometry, John Wiley & Son, 1976

35. Narayanan C.R., Natu A.A., Triterpene Acids of Indian Clove Buds, Phytochemistry, *13*, 1999-2000, 1974

36. Saito Y., Kimura Y., Sakamoto T., Studies on the antioxidative properties of spices. III The antioxidative effects of petroleum ether soluble and insoluble fractions from spices, through Chem. Abstr. *87*, 150314r, 1977

37. Vösgen B., Kiok G., Herrmann K., Flavonoglykoside von Pfeffer (*Piper nigrum* L.), Gewürznelken (*Syzygium aromaticum* (L.) Merr. et Perry) und Piment (Pimenta dioica (L.) Merr.), Z. Lebensm. Unters. Forsch., 170, 204-207, 1980

38. IFRA - Code of practice. Isogenol monograph. May 1980, last amendment June 1992

39. Recommendations concerning undesirable active principles, 3.11, 28th meeting Committee of Experts on Cosmetic Products, Rome, 3-7 November 1997, Council of Europe

40. Recommendations concerning undesirable active principles, 3.16, 28th meeting Committee of Experts on Cosmetic Products, Rome, 3-7 November 1997, Council of Europe

41. OAB 9

42. Ph Helv. VII

43. DAB 9

44. BP '93

45. FU IX

Taraxacum officinale

Botanical name[1]	*Taraxacum officinale* Weber
Botanical synonyms[2]	*Leontodon taraxacum* L., *Taraxacum dens-leonis* Desf., *Taraxacum taraxacum* Karst., *Taraxacum vulgare* Schrank
Botanical family	Asteraceae
Common names	Dandelion (English) Paardebloem (Dutch) Voikukka (Finnish) Pissenlit (French) Lowenzahn (German) Tarassaco (Italian) Løvetann (Norwegian) Amargón (Spanish) Naskros (Swedish)
EU INCI name[3]	*Taraxacum officinale*
CTFA INCI name[4]	Dandelion (*Taraxacum officinale*) extract Dandelion (*Taraxacum officinale*) root

CAS number	68990-74-9 84775-55-3
EINECS number	273-624-6
Parts used	Roots and rhizomes

Important constituents including active principles[7, 12, 15]

- Inulin (up to 40%)[11, 14]
- Triterpenes (taraxol, taraxerol, taraxasterol, φ-taraxasterol, β-amyrin)
- Flavonoids (luteolin-7-glucoside, apigenin-7-glucoside)
- Vitamins
- Phenol acids (caffeic and p-hydroxyphenylacetic acids) Tannins (phlobapenes)
- Phytosterols (stigmasterol, β-sitosterol, campesterol, homoandrosterol, homotaraxasterol)
- Sesquiterpene lactones
- Fatty acids (linolenic, linoleic, melissic, oleic and palmitic acids)
- Lactucopicrin
- Amino acids (choline)
- Levulin
- Sugars (fructose, glucose, sucrose) (up to 18%)[15]
- Polyalcohol (mannitol)

                                             – Pectins up to 8%

                                             – Proteins

                                             – Gum resin

                                             – Mineral salts (mainly potassium)

Preparation

1) Fluid aqueous extract E/D = 1:1
2) Dried aqueous extract E/D = 1: 5
3) Hydroalcoholic tincture T/D = 5:1

Manufacturing process

1) Maceration of roots and rhizomes with water and concentration under vacuum to final E/D ratio 1:1.
2) Maceration of roots and rhizomes with water and concentration under vacuum to dryness.
3) Maceration of roots and rhizomes with alcohol 20%.

Examples of specifications -

Intended cosmetic effects and used concentration in cosmetic products
Astringent, refreshing, tonic, lightening, purifying

Other possible effects

Anti-inflammatory, freckle lightening (traditional use) (Taraxasterol)[17, 21]

Anti-inflammatory activity reported against TPA together with antimicrobial activity against *Staphylococcus aureus*.

Main toxicological data[10]

LD_{50} i.p. in mice: 36.6 g/kg

Contact dermatitis to dandelion extracts has been reported[20, 23]

Databases used

CA Search 1967-96, Medline 1966-96, Embase 1974-96, Reg. Tox. Eff. Chem. Sub., Naprelert, Toxline, Cosmet

Keywords

Taraxacum officinale, Dandelion

Evaluation and remarks

Cat. B

General references

1. Index Kewensis, Clarendon Press
2. Penso G., Index Plantarum Medicinalium Totius Mundi Eorumque Synonymorum, OEMF, 1983
3. European Commission Decision 96/335/EC of 8 May 1996, Official Journal of the European Community No. L132 of 1 June 1996
4. International Cosmetic Ingredient Dictionary 6th ed., CTFA, 2, 1995
5. Benigni R., Capra C., Cattorini P.E., Piante Medicinali chimica farmacologia e terapia, Inverni & Della Beffa, 2, 1593-1599, 1964
6. Council of Europe, Flavouring substances and natural sources of flavourings, 3rd ed Maisonneuve, (447, N2), 1981
7. Leung A.Y., Foster S., Encyclopedia of common natural ingredients, Wiley & Son Publ., 205-207, 1996
8. Martindale 31st ed., The Royal Pharmaceutical Society, 1996
9. Merck Index 12th ed., Merck & Co. Inc., 1996
10. Monograph Taraxaci radix (Dandelion root), European Scientific Cooperative for Phytoterapy (ESCOP), 1996

11. Monograph Taraxaci radix cum herba, Bundesanzeiger, No. 228 (Dec 5, through Le monografie tedesche, Studio Edizioni, *3*, 1995

12. Newall C., Anderson L., Phillipson J.D., Herbal Medicines a guide for health care professionals, The Pharmaceutical Press, 96-97, 1996

13. Paris R.R., Moyse H., Matière Médicale, Masson, *3*, 429, 1981

14. Proserpio G., Martelli A., Patri G.F., Elementi di fitocosmesi, Sepem, *2*, 1982

15. Van Hellemont J., Compendium de Phytotherapie, APB, 390-392, 1986

16. Wichtl M., Teedrogen, WVG, 315-318, 1989

Specific references

17. Akihisa T., Yasukawa K., Oinuma H., Kasahara Y., Yamanouchi S., Takido M., Kumaki K., Tamura T., Triterpene alcohols from the flowers of compositae and their Anti-inflammatory effects, Phytochemistry, *43*, 6, 1255-1260, 1996

18. Grauds C., Dandelion: common weed and herbal remedy, Pharm. Times *62*, 80-, 1996

19. Heath H.B., Herbs -their use in cosmetics and toiletries, Cosm: and Toil., *92*, 19-24, 1977

20. Nater J.P., De Groot A.C., Unwanted effects of cosmetics and drugs used in dermatology, Excerpta Medica, 314, 321, 1983

21. Villarreal M.L., Alvarez L., Alonso D., Navarro V., Garcia P., Delgado G., Cytotoxic and antimicrobial screening of selected terpenoids from Asteraceae species, J. Ethnopharmacol, *42*, 1, 25-29,1994

22. Yasukawa K., Akihisa T., Oinuma H., Kaminaga T., Kanno H., Kasahara Y., Tamura T., Kumaki K., Yamanouchi S., Takido M., Inhibitory effect of taraxastane-type triterpenes on tumor promotion by 12-o-tetradecanoylphorbol-13-acetate (TPA) in two-strage carcinogenesis in mouse skin, Oncology, *53*, 4, 341-344, 1996

23. Recommendations concerning undesirable active principles, 3.1, 28th meeting Committee of Experts on Cosmetic Products, Rome, 3-7 November 1997, Council of Europe.

24. DAC '86

25. OAB '81

26. BHP 1990

27. BPC 1949

Terminalia sericea

Botanical name[1].	*Terminalia sericea* Burk.
Botanical synonyms[1]	*Terminalia sericea* DC.
Botanical family	Combretaceae
Common names	Terminalia sericea (English)
	Badamier (French)
	Terminalia sericea (Norwegian)
EU INCI name[2]	*Terminalia sericea*
CTFA INCI name[3]	*Terminalia sericea* extract

CAS number	90131-49-0
	55306-04-2 (sericoside)
EINECS number	290-360-7
	259-586-3 (sericoside)
Parts used	Bark and roots

Important constituents including active principles[5]

- Triterpene saponins (sericoside (1.2%)[9], arjunglucoside, arjune-tine) and genins (sericic acid (0.05%), arjungenin, arjunic acid)
- Amino acids (lysine, serine, aspartic acid, glycine, threonine and valine)
- Hydroxystilbene glycoside (resveratrol 3-O-rutinoside)[4]
- Ellagic acid
- Tannins
- Sugars

Preparation	Purified dry extract (Sericoside)
Manufacturing process	Percolation with alcohol 80% and purification by n-butanol.
Examples of specifications	Assay: not less than 70%
	Sulphated ash: less than 1%
	Water: less than 5%

Intended cosmetic effects and used concentration in cosmetic products

Smoothing, soothing

Up to 2% in products for sensitive skin and mucosae, swollen and bleeding gums, eye puffiness, anti-wrinkles or anti-stretch marks, after-sun, after-shave, after depilation

Other possible effects

Granulation promoting agent, anti-inflammatory, healing, anti-oedema, heavy legs, anti-fungal[7].

Main toxicological data	(sericoside)[8]

LD_{50} oral in rats: > 5 000 mg/kg
LD_{50} i.p. in rats: > 2 000 mg/kg
Primary skin irritation in rabbits: non-irritant
Acute eye irritation in rabbits: non-irritant
Sensibilisation in guinea pigs: non-sensitising
Sensibilisation in humans (3% gel): non-sensitising

(total extract)[5]
LD_{50} i.p. in rats: 200 mg/kg

Databases used

CA Search 1967-96, Medline 1966-96, Embase 1974-96, Reg. Tox. Eff. Chem. Sub.

Keywords

Terminalia sericea

Evaluation and remarks

Cat. A

General references

1. Index Kewensis, Clarendon Press
2. European Commission Decision 96/335/EC of 8 May 1996, Official Journal of the European Community No. L132 of 1 June 1996
3. International Cosmetic Ingredient Dictionary 6th ed., CTFA, *2*, 1995

Specific references

4. Bombardelli E., Martinelli E.M., Mustich G., Plants of Mozambique. A new Hydroxystilbene glycoside from Terminalia sericea, Fitoterapia, *46*, 199, 1975
5. Bombardelli E., Crippa F., Pifferi G., Sericoside, a new glucoside in functional cosmetics, Preprints of XIVth IFSCC Congress, Barcellona, 1986
6. Hegnauer R., Chemotaxonomie der Pflanzen, Birkhauser, 8, 254- 260, 1989
7. Hess S.C., Brum R.L., Honda N.K. et al, Anti-fungal activity of Sericic Acid, Fitoterapia, *66*, 6, 549-550, 1995
8. Indena's reports
9. Pifferi G., Zini G.F. Cristoni A., Sericoside: Anti-inflammatory Activity and Occurrence in Plants of the Terminalia genus, Phytochemical Society of Europe, Symposium "Biologically Active Natural Products", Lausanne, 1986

Tropaeolum majus

Botanical name[1]	*Tropaeolum majus* L.
Botanical synonyms	-
Botanical family	Tropaeolaceae
Common names	Indian cress (English)
	Oostindische kers (Dutch)
	Koristekrassi (Finnish)
	Capucine (French)
	Kapuzinerkresse (German)
	Nasturzio d'India (Italian)
	Blomkarse (Norwegian)
	Capuchina (Spanish)
	Krasse (Swedish)
EU INCI name[2]	*Tropaeolum majus*
CTFA INCI name[3]	Indian cress (*Tropaeolum majus*) extract

CAS number	84625-49-0
EINECS number	283-419-3
Parts used	Flowers, leaves and stems

Important constituents including active principles[5, 10]
- Essential oil (0.03%)[5]:
  Sulphurated heteroside (glucotropaeoline releasing benzyl-isothiocyanate)[12]
- Flavonoids (isoquercitrin, isoquercitroside, quercetin-3-triglucoside, kaempferol-glucoside, pelargonidin-3-bioside, pelargonidin-3-sophoroside)
- Xanthophyll (lutein, zeaxanthin)
- Polyene hydrocarbon (phytofluene)
- Amino acids
- Proteins
- Vitamin C
- Fatty acids (erucic, linoleic, linolenic and gondoic acids)
- Mineral salts

Preparation[10]	Hydroglycolic extract
Manufacturing process[10]	Percolation of fresh aerial part with propylene glycol 50% to final E/D ratio 1:1

Examples of specifications[10.]   pH: 5.0 to 6.5
Relative density at 20°C: 1.035 to 1.045
Refractive index at 20°C: 1.385 to 1.395
Dry residue: 0.30 to 1.00%
Heavy metals: ≤ 5 ppm

Intended cosmetic effects and used concentration in cosmetic products
Tonic, purifying agent, antidandruff
Up to 5% in cleansing lotions, creams, gels and bath products for oily and impure skin
Up to 10% in shampoos for oily scalp, hair-care products, products to prevent hair loss (traditional use)

Other possible effects   Antimicrobial, rubifacient[4.], anti-acnes
Benzyl-isothiocyanate is reported to show antitumoral activity[11.]

Main toxicological data   Allergenicity data are reported.[4.] Not to be used for babies or small children.[4.]
Primary skin irritation in rabbits: non-irritant [15.]
Acute eye irritation in rabbits: non-irritant[15.]

Databases used   CA Search 1967-95, Medline 1966-95, Embase 1974-95, Ref. Tox. Eff. Chem. Sub., Biosis, Toxline, Kosmet, Cancerlit

Keywords   *Tropaeolum majus*

Evaluation and remarks   **Cat. A (Hydroglycolic extract) but not to be used on children under 10**

General references
1. Index Kewensis, Clarendon Press
2. European Commission Decision 96/335/EC of 8 May 1996, Official Journal of the European Community No. L132 of 1 June 1996
3. International Cosmetic Ingredient Dictionary 6th ed., CTFA, 1995
4. Monographs, Bundesanzeiger Tropaeolum majus, n 162 (Ago. 29, 1992), through Le monografie tedesche, Studio Edizioni, *4*, 1996
5. Paris R.R., Moyse H., Matière Médicale, Masson, 2nd ed, *2*, 218-219, 1981
6. Proserpio G., Martelli A., Patri G.F., Elementi di fitocosmesi, Sepem, *2*, 568, 1983
7. Van Hellemont J., Compendium de Phytotherapie, APB, 408-409, 1986

Specific references
8. Beckstrom-Sternberg SM, Duke J.A. "The Phytochemical Database"
9. Carlson K.D., Kleiman R., Chemical survey and erucic acid content of commercial varieties of nasturtium, *Tropeolum maius* L., JAOCS, *70*, 11, 1145-1148, 1993
10. Franz G., Regensburg, Kapuzinerkresse (*Tropeolum maius* L.), Zeitschrift für Phyto therapie 17, 255-262, 1996

11. Kjaer A., the distribution of sulphur compounds, Chemical plant taxonomy, Swain ed., T. London Academic press, 453, 1963
12. Indena Product Specification
13. Pintão A.M.,Pais M.S.S., Coley H., Kelland L.R. and Judson R., In vitro and in vivo Antitumor Activity of Benzyl Isothiocyanate: a Natural Product from Tropaeolum majus, Planta medica, *61*, 233-236, 1995
14. Radwan S.S., Localization of Lipids Containig (Z)-11-Eicosenoic Acid and (Z)-13-Docosenoic acid in Tropaeolum majus, Phytochemistry, *15*, 1727-1729, 1976
15. Indena's reports

Tussilago farfara

Botanical name[1]	*Tussilago farfara* L.
Botanical synonyms[1]	*Tussilago vulgaris* Lam.
Botanical family	Asteraceae
Common names	Coltsfoot (English)
	Klein Hoefblad (Dutch)
	Leskenlehti (Finnish)
	Pas d'âne, tussilage (French)
	Kleiner Huflattich (German)
	Farfaro (Italian)
	Hestehov (Norwegian)
	Tusílago (Spanish)
	Hästhov (Swedish)
EU INCI name[2]	*Tussilago farfara*
CTFA INCI name[3]	Coltsfoot (*Tussilago farfara*) extract
	Coltsfoot (*Tussilago farfara*) leaf extract

CAS number	84625-50-3
EINECS number	283-420-9
Parts used	Leaves and flowers, roots (sometimes)

Important constituents including active principles[10, 14]

- Essential oil
- Flavonoids (rutoside 0.36% (flowers)[10], hyperoside 0.8% (leaves)[10], quercetin glucosides, 0.28% (flowers)[10], spiracoside, avicularoside, kaempferol-3-glucoside, kaempferol-3-arabinoside)
- Coumarins (esculetin)
- Phenol acids (caffeic, ferulic, p-hydroxybenzoic acid, caffeoyltartaric, gallic, tannic)
- Polysaccharides (pectines and inulin 8.2% (leaves)[14])
- Triterpene alcohols (arnidiol, faradiol)
- Sesquiterpenes (notonipetranone, tussilagone)[31]
- Triterpenes (a- and b-amyrine)
- Phytosterols (campesterol, b-sitosterol, taraxasterol)
- Tannins 17% (leaves)[14]
- Fatty acids
- Organic acids (malic and tartaric)
- Pirrolizidine alkaloids (neosenkirkine, senkirkine 0.01%[18], tussilagine, isotussilagine senecionine, integerrimine, seneciphylline)

Preparation

1) Aqueous dry extract
2) Hydroalcoholic extract E/D = 1:1
3) Hydroglycolic extract[4]

Manufacturing process

1) Percolation with water and concentration under vacuum to dryness ratio
2) Percolation with alcohol 30% and concentration under vacuum to final E/D ratio 1:1
3) Percolation with propylene glycol 50% from flowers

Examples of specifications

1)[4] Heavy metals: not more than 20 ppm
Arsenic: not more than 2 ppm
Residue on evaporation: not more than 2%

Intended cosmetic effects and used concentration in cosmetic products

Smoothing, soothing, astringent, purifying
Products for impure, oily, sensitive and chapped skin, products for oily scalp

Other possible effects

Antibacterial[30], granulation-promoting agent[10]

Main toxicological data

(aqueous extract)[22]
LD_{50} oral in mice: > 5000mg/kg
LD_{50} i.p. in mice: > 5000 mg/kg
TDL_0 oral in rats: 4 800 g/kg (carcinogenic liver-tumors) [RTECS]

(polyphenol fraction)[22]
LD_{50} oral in mice: > 5000mg/kg
LD_{50} i.p. in mice: > 5 000 mg/kg

(Pyrrolizidine alkaloids)
Pyrrolizidin alkaloids present in Tussilago farfara include senkirkine, tusilagine and senecionine. Feeding studies with the flowers buds (8% and 16% of the diet for 600 days) increases occurrence of liver carcinomas in rats.[27, 45] Senkirkine is mutagenic in several test systems [17, 19, 20, 42] and senecionine is also suspected of being mutagenic [17, 20, 24].

The toxic effects of pyrrolizidine alkaloids are due to activation in the liver where metabolism by mixed-function oxidases leads to pyrrolic dehydro-alkaloids which are reactive alkylating agents. The carcinogenic activity of pyrrolizidine alkaloids appears to parallel their mutagenic behaviour[44].

(Kaempferol)[23, 34]
Tussilago components such as kaempferol are mutagenic

(According to the Commission E monograph, the use of Tussilago farfara is not recommended because of lack of documentation)[10]

Databases used

CA Search 1967-95, Medline 1966-95, Embase 1974-95, Ref. Tox. Eff. Chem. Sub., HSDE, Cab Plant, Emtox, CCRIS, IPA, Napralert, Toxline, Cosmet

Keywords

Tussilago farfara, coltsfoot

Evaluation and remarks   Cat. C

General references

1. Index Kewensis, Clarendon Press
2. European Commission Decision 96/335/EC of 8 May 1996, Official Journal of the European Community No. L132 of 1 June 1996
3. International Cosmetic Ingredient Dictionary 6th ed., CTFA, *1*, 1995
4. Comprehensive Licensing Standards of Cosmetics by Category, Yakuji Nippo Ltd. *2*, 431, 1987
5. Council of Europe, Flavouring substances and natural sources of flavourings 3rd ed., Maisonneuve, (463, N4), 1981
6. Grieve M., A modern herbal, Barnes & Noble Books, *1*, 212-214, 1996
7. The Japanese Cosmetic Ingredients Codex, Yakuji Nippo, Ltd., 167-168, 1993
8. Martindale 31st ed., The Royal Pharmaceutical Society, 1996
9. Merck Index 12th ed., Merck & Co. Inc., 1996
10. Monograph Farfarae flos, Farfarae herba, Farfarae radix and Farfarae folium, Bundesanzeiger, No. 138 (July 27, 1990) through Le monografie tedesche, Studio Edizioni, 4, 1996
11. Newall C., Anderson L., Phillipson J.D., Herbal Medicines a guide for health care professionals, The Pharmaceutical Press, 85-86, 1996
12. Paris R.R., Moyse H., Matière Médicale, Masson, *3*, 462-463, 1971-
13. Proserpio G., Martelli A., Patri G.F., Elementi di fitocosmesi, Sepem, I, 1982
14. Van Hellemont J., Compendium de Phytotherapie, APB, 410-411, 1986
15. Wichtl M., Teedrogen, WVG, 246-248, 1989

Specific references

16. Akras, Product specification
17. Austrian delegation data sheets, April 1996
18. Borka, Laszlo, Onshuus, Inger, Senkirkine content Is the leaves of Tussilago farfara L.through Chem. Abstr, *92*, 3225n, 1980
19. Candrian U., Lüthy J., Graf U., Schlatter Ch., Mutagenic activity of pyrrolizidine alkaloids seneciphylline and senkirkine in drosophila and their transfer into rat milk, Fd. Chem. Toxic., I, 3, 223-225, 1984
20. Danninger T., Hagermann U., Schmidt V., Schonhofer P.S., Pharm. Ztg., 128, 289-303, 1983
21. De Vincenzi M., Dessi M.R., Botanical flavouring substances used in foods: proposal of classification *Tussilago farfara* L., Fitoterapia, I, 1, 1991
22. Didry N., Pinkas M., Torck M.and Dubreuil L., Sur la composition chimique et l'activité du Tussilage, Ann. Pharm. Fr., *40*, 1, 75-80, 1982
23. Fukuoka M., Kuroyanagi M. et al., Chemical and Toxicological Studies on Brancken Fern, Pteridium Aquilinum var.

Latiusculum. VI. Surveys on Bracken Constituents by Mutagen Test, J. Pharm. Dyn. *1*, 324-331, 1978

24. Green C.E., Segall H.J., Byard J.L., Metabolism, Cytotoxicity and Genotoxicity of the Pyrrolizidine Alkaloid Senencionine in Primary Cultures of Rat Hepatocytes, Toxicol Appl. Pharmacol., *60*, 176-185, 1981

25. Hagers, Handbuch der pharmazeutischen Praxis, Springer Verlag, Auflage, *6*, 1016-1023, 1993

26. Heath H.B., Herbs-their use in cosmetics and toiletries, Cosm. and Toil., *92*, 19-24, 1977

27. Hirono I, Mori H., Culvenor C.C.J., Carcinogenic activity of Coltsfoot, GANN *67*, 125-129, 1976

28. Hoppe H. A., Drogenkunde, W. de Gruyter, 8th ed., 1134-1137, 1975

29. Hoppe H. A., Drogenkunde, W. de Gruyter, 305-306, 1981

30. Izzo A.A., Di Carlo G. et al., Biological screening of Italian medicinal plants for antibacterial activity, Phyto ther. Res., *9*, 281-286, 1995

31. Kikuchi M., Suzuki N., Studies on the constituents of Tussilago farfara L. Structure of new sesquiterpenoids isolated from the flower buds, Chem, Pharm.Bull. *40*, 10, 2753-2755, 1992

32. Lewis R.J., Sax's Dangerous Properties of Industrial Materials, 8th ed.

33. Marquardt H., Lehrbuch der Toxikologie, BI Wissenschaftsverlag, 677f, 1995

34. Nagao M., Yahagi T., Sugimura T., Differences in Effects of Norharman with Various Classes of Chemical Mutagens and Amount of S-9, Biochem. Byophys. Res. Comm., *83*, 373-378, 1978

35. Nater J.P., De Groot A.C., Unwanted effects of cosmetics and drugs used in dermatology, Excerpta Medica, 314,321, 1983

36. Nater J.P., De Groot A.C., Unwanted effects of cosmetics and drugs used in dermatology, Elsevier, 2nd ed., 385, 1994

37. Plantapharm, Fax vom, 16.11.1995

38. Physiological Efficacy and Harmlessness of Cosmetic Hair Lotions, Relata Technica 30, 45-46, 1982

39. Steinegger E., Hansel R., Lehrburch der Pharmakognosie, Springer-Lehrburch, 3. Auflage, 100-101, 1972; 5. Auflage, 127, 1994

40. Takanashi H., Umeda M., Hirono I., Chromosomal Aberrations and Mutation in Cultured Mammalian Cells Induced by Pyrrolizidine Alkaloids, Mutat. Res. 78, 67-77, 1980

41. Williams G.M., Mori H., Genotoxicity of Pyrrolizidine Alkaloids in the Hepatocyte Primary Culture/DNA- Repair Test, Mutat. Res., 79, 1, 1980

42. Yamanaka H., Nagao M. et al., Mutagenicity of Pyrrolizidine Alkaloids in the Salmonella/Mammalian-Microsome Test, Mutat. Res., 68, 211-216, 1979

43. Zepernick, Longhammer, Ludcke, Lexikon der offiziellen Arzneipflanzen, 423-424, 1984
44. Recommendations concerning undesirable active principles, 3.15, 28th meeting Committee of Experts on Cosmetic Products, Rome, 3-7 November 1997, Council of Europe
45. IARC Monograph 10, 125, 1976
46. - DAB 10
47. - OAB '90
48. - Helv. VII
49. - Pr. Fr. VIII
50. - Ph. Helv. VII
51. - Br. Herb. Ph. '83

Usnea spp.

Botanical name	*Usnea barbata* (L.) Wigg. (is the main species used)
Botanical synonyms	-
Botanical family	Usneaceae
Common names	Lichen (English)
	Lichen chevelu (French)
	Bartflechten (German)
	Lichene (Italian)
	Skjegglav (Norwegian)
	Serra (Spanish)
	Skägglav (Swedish)
EU INCI name[1]	*Usnea barbata*
	Usnic acid
CTFA INCI name[2]	Lichen (*Usnea barbata*) extract
	Usnic acid

CAS number	84696-53-7 (*Usnea barbata*)
	125-46-2 (usnic acid)
EINECS number	283-658-3 (*Usnea barbata*)
	204-740-7 (usnic acid)
Parts used	Thallus

Important constituents including active principles[6]

– Lichen acids (furane derivatives: usnic acid up to 4%[6]; depsidones: psoromic and demethylpsoromic acids[12])

– Aromatic acids

– Aliphatic acids

– Polisaccharides (lichenin and isolichenin)[4]

– Mineral salts

Preparation	1) Usnic acid
	2) Extract
Manufacturing process	1) Extraction with ethanol and crystallisation
Examples of specifications	1) Melting point: 204°C
	Specific optical rotation at 16°C: (c=0.7 in $CHCL_3$): + 509.4°

Intended cosmetic effects and used concentration in cosmetic products

Soothing, purifying, deodorant, antidandruff

Up to 0.5% in detergents and in deodorant. In toothpastes as plaque inhibitor

Other possible effects

Anti-microbial, analgesic, antipyretic, anti-inflammatory[7], immuno-stimulant

Main toxicological data [RTECS]

(Usnic acid):

LD_{50} oral in rabbits: > 500 mg/kg

LD_{50} i.v. in mice: 25 mg/kg

LD_{50} i.v. in rats and rabbits: 30 mg/kg

LD_{50} i.v. in dogs: 40 mg/kg

LD_{50} subcutaneous in mice: 700 mg/kg

LD_{50} oral mice: 515 mg/kg

LD_{50} oral rats: 220 mg/kg

Weakly irritant on rabbit skin

Rabbit eye test: 0.1 ml of a 12.5% solution was tolerated without irritation; 25% solution provoked a slight and reversible oedema; 50% solution provoked a reversible erythema

Maximisation test on guinea-pigs: no sensitisation

Genotoxicity tests: 2 positive results, but of dubious relevance: Rat-kangaroo cell cultures showed chromosomal anomalies and mitotic inhibition study of 1970; unusual test system and therefore difficult to interpret)

DNA-cell binding test was positive if lysozyme was added

Ames-test: up to 200 mg/plate negatif, with and without activation

Sensitisation[13]: in guinea-pigs and humans no evidence

(Lichenin)[4]

Exhibits antineoplastic activity

(Hydroalcoholic tincture T:D = 10:1)[7]

LD_{50} oral mice: no mortality recorded

LD_{50} i.p. in mice: 22.53 g/kg b. w.

LD_{50} i.v. in mice: 7.43 g/kg b.w.

Databases used

CA Search 1967-95, Medline, 1966-95, Embase 1974-95, Reg. Tox. Eff. Chem. Sub.

Keywords

Usnea

Evaluation and remarks

Cat. B (usnic acid; extract)

Usnic acid is a relatively powerful antibiotic that used to be on sale in pharmacies in the form of dermatological preparations. It is produced by a fungus living in a symbiosis in lichen. It would appear to have significant toxic cell effects, whence the need for further information.

General references

1. European Commission Decision 96/335/EC of 8 May 1996, Official Journal of the European Community No. L132 of 1 June 1996

Specific references

2. International Cosmetic Ingredient Dictionary 6th ed., CTFA, *1, 2*, 1995
3. Martindale 31st ed., The Royal Pharmaceutical Society, 1996
4. Merck Index 12th ed., Merck & Co. Inc., 1996
5. Paris R.R., Moyse H., Matière Médicale 12nd ed., Masson, *1*, 367, 1976
6. CE data sheet ref.: CD-P-SP(94) 34, pt. 5 7.1 (record 23rd session, Oct.1994
7. Dobrescu D. et al., Contributions to the complex study of some lichens- *Usnea* genus. Pharmacological studies on Usnea barbata and *Usnea hirta* species, Rom. J. Physiol., *30*, 1-2, 101-107, 1993
8. Fontana M., Proserpio G., L'acido usnico come preservante naturale, deodorante e dermopurificante nei sistemi cosmetici, EPPOS 315-336, 1974
9. Garty J., Ammann K., The amounts of Ni, Cr, Zn, Pb, Cu, Fe and Mn in some lichens growing in Switzerland, Environmental and Experimental Botany *27*, 2 127-138, 1987
10. Gibaja Oviedo S., Carrillo G.C., Química de Líquenes II. Estudio de Usnea barbata (L) Wigg., Boll. de la Sociedad Química del Perú, 88-90,
11. Iacomini M., Gorin P.A.J., Baron M. et al., Novel d-glucans obtained by dimethylsulfoxide extraction of lichens *Letharia vulpina, Actinogyra muehlenbergii* and an *Usnea* Sp, Carbohydrate Research, *176*, 117-126, 1988
12. Keogh M., 2'-o-demethylpsoromic acid from Usnea sp, Phytochemistry, *15*, 1801, 1976
13. Mitchell J.C. and Maibach H.I., Sensitising capacity of usnic acid derived from lichenised fungi, Acta derm.-venereol. 49, 498-500, 1969
14. Okuyama E., Umeyama K., Kinoshita Y. and Yamamoto Y., Usnic Acid and diffractaic acid as analgesic and antipyretic components of Usnea diffacta, Planta Med., *61*, 113-115, 1995
15. Orissa Drebing GmbH, Deodorising cosmetic composition, Deutsches Patentamt, Cl. A 61 K 7-32, 24 April 1975
16. Proserpio G., Antimicrobici cutanei nei prodotti cosmetici antiforfora deodoranti- dermopurificanti, Boll. Chim. Farm., 124, 347-355, 1985
17. Seifert P., Bertrand C., Usnic acid- Natural preservation from lichen, SOFW- Journal *121*, 7, 480- 485, 1995
18. Grievson M., Barber J. And Huting A.L.L., Natural Ingredients in Cosmetics, 101-109, May 23, 1989

Viscum album

Botanical name[1]	*Viscum album* L., *Viscum album* L. ssp. *abietis* Beck, *Viscum album* L. ssp. *coloratum* Kom., *Viscum album* L. ssp. *laxum* Fiek., *Viscum album* L. ssp. *platyspermum* Kell.
Botanical synonyms	-
Botanical family	Viscaceae
Common names	Mistletoe (English) Maretak (Dutch) Misteli (Finnish) Gui (French) Mistel (German) Vischio (Italian) Misteltein (Norwegian) Liga (Spanish) Mistel (Swedish)
EU INCI name[2]	Viscum album
CTFA INCI name[3]	Mistletoe (*Viscum album*) Mistletoe (*Viscum album*) extract Mistletoe (*Viscum album*) leaf extract

CAS number	84929-55-5 8031-76-3 (extract)
EINECS number	284-538-3
Parts used	Berries, leaves and twigs

Important constituents including active principles[4, 10]
- Polypeptides (viscotoxin A_2, A_3, B, PS_1) 0.1%[9]
- Lectins (viscumin, mistelectin I, II, III)
- Proteins
  Flavonoids (flavonol, flavonone and chalcone derivatives)
- Phenol acids (caffeic and derivatives, gentisic, ferulic, myristic, p-hydroxybenzoic, p-hydroxyphenylacetic, protocatechuic, shikimic, sinapic, quinic and vanillic acids)
- Polyalcohols (mannitol, inositol 2%[9], quebrachitol, pinitol, vis-cumitol, dulcitol, xylitol, quercitol)
- Triterpene saponins and relevant aglycones (β-amyrine, lupeol, oleanolic, betulinic, ursolic acids)
- Amines (choline, acetylcholine, β-phenylethyalanine, tyramine, histamine, propionylcholine)

- Amino acids (g-aminobutiric acid)
- Phenylpropanes (syringine)
- Phytosterols (β-sitosterol, dihydro-β-sitosterol, stigmasterol, sterol A, phytosterol glucoside)
- Fatty acids (oleic and palmitic acids)
- Tannins
- Polysaccharides (pectins, hemicellulose, starch, viscin)
- Sugars (fructose, glucose, raffinose, sucrose)

Preparation

1) Aqueous dry extract
2) Hydroalcoholic extract
3) Hydroglycolic extract

Manufacturing process

1) Percolation with water and concentration under vacuum to dryness
2) Percolation with alcohol 35% and concentration to final E/D ratio 1:1
3) Percolation with propylene glycol 45% and concentration to final E/D ratio 4:1

Examples of specifications[14]

1) Syringin and syringinapiosylglucoside: 0.6%
   Viscumin: 145 to 920 mg/ml

Intended cosmetic effects and used concentration in cosmetic products

Soothing, anti-itching

Other possible effects

Anti-inflammatory, hypotensive, cytostatic, traditionally used on ulcers and sores

Main toxicological data

(extract)[(RTECS),23]
LD_{50} i.p. in mice: 250 mg/kg
LD_{50} i.v. in mice: 235 µg /Kg

(viscotoxin A)[(RTECS)]
LD_{50} i.p. in mice: 780 µg/kg.
Cytotoxic to HeLa/KB cells IC_{50}: 0.2 to 1.7 mg/ml

(viscumin)
LD_{50} i.v. in mice: 2.4 µg/kg.
Inhibits protein synthetase in rabbit reticulocytes lysate and has cytotoxic effect in man[23]

(mistelectin I, II and III)
Induction of apoptosis in isolated human lymphocytes[15]
Acute toxicity of ML I in the mouse is very high and related to effects on liver enzymes (0.6 µg/kg) increased drastically liver phosphatase[16]

(polysaccharide fraction)
LD_{50} i.p. in mice: >2250 mg/kg

Databases used

CA Search 1980-1995, Medline 1980-1995, Embase 1980-1995, Ref. Tox. Eff. Chem. Sub., Toxline, Toxbio, IPA, ECDIN, EMTOX , Cosmet, Napralert

Keywords

Viscum album, Mistletoe

Evaluation and remarks

Cat. C (aqueous dry extract; hydroalcoholic extract; hydroglycolic extract)

Given the level of cytotoxicity of some of the constituents, mistletoe preparations should not be accepted unless it can be proved that they are completely harmless.

General references

1. Index Kewensis, Clarendon Press
2. European Commission Decision 96/335/EC of 8 May 1996, Official Journal of the European Community No. L132 of 1 June 1996
3. International Cosmetic Ingredient Dictionary 6th ed., CTFA, *1*, 1995
4. Benigni R., Capra C., Cattorini P.E., Piante Medicinali chimica farmacologia e terapia, Inverni & Della Beffa, *2*, 1760-1782, 1964
5. Council of Europe, Flavouring substances and natural sources of flavourings 3rd ed., Maisonneuve, (484,N3), 1981
6. Grieve M., A modern herbal, Barnes & Noble Books, *2*, 547-548, 1996
7. Martindale 31st ed., The Royal Pharmaceutical Society, 1996
8. Monograph Visci albi herba, Bundesanzeiger, n. 228 (Dec 05, 1984) and Visci albi fructus n. 128 (July 14, 1993) through Le monografie tedesche, Studio Edizioni, *4*, 1996
9. Newall C., Anderson L., Phillipson J.D., Herbal Medicines a guide for health care professionals, The Pharmaceutical Press, 193-196, 1996
10. Paris R.R., Moyse H., Matière Médicale 2nd ed., Masson, *2*, 108-109, 1981
11. Van Hellemont J., Compendium de Phytotherapie, APB, 428-430, 1986
12. Wichtl M., Teedrogen, WVG, 343-345, 1989

Specific references

13. Akras, Datenkennblatt, 16.11.1995
14. Austrian delegation data sheet, November 1995
15. Bussing A., Suzart K., Bergmann J., Pfuller U., Schietzel M., Schweizer K., Induction of apoptosis in human lymphocytes treated with Viscum album L. is mediated by the mistletoe lectins, Cancer Lett, *99*, 1, 59-72, 1996
16. Gossrau R. and Franz H., Histochemical response of mice to mistletoe lectin I (ML I) from the toxic drug, Histochemistry, *94*, 5, 531-537, 1990
17. Franz H., Mistletoe lectins and their A and B chains, Oncology, *43*, 1s, 23-34, 1986
18. Hagers, Handbuch der pharmazeutischen Praxis, Springer Verlag, Auflage, 483, 1993
19. Hoppe H. A., Drogenkunde, W. de Gruyter, 8th ed, 1134-1137, 1975
20. Hoppe H. A., Drogenkunde, W. de Gruyter, 305-306, 1981
21. Lewis R.J., Sax's Dangerous Properties of Industrial Materials, 8th ed.

22. Nater J.P., De Groot A.C., Unwanted effects of cosmetics and drugs used in dermatology, Elsevier, 2nd ed., 385-388; 3rd ed., 694, 1994
23. Olsnes S., Stirpe F., Sandvig K., Pihl A., Isolation and Characterization of Viscumin, a toxic Lectin from Viscum album L. (Mistletoe) J. Biol. Chem., *257*, 22,13263-13270, 1982
24. Plantapharm, Datenkennblatt, 16.11.1995
25. Steinegger E., Hansel R., Lehrburch der Pharmakognosie, Springer
26. Br. Herb. Ph. '83
27. DAB 10
28. DAC '86
29. OAB '83
30. Ph. Helv. VII
31. Ph. Fr. VIII
32. Erg. B. 6

Vitis vinifera

Botanical name[1]	*Vitis vinifera* L.
Botanical synonyms	-
Botanical family	Vitaceae
Common names	Grape (English) Wijnstok (Dutch) Viiniköynnös (Finnish) Vigne (French) Weinrebe (German) Vite (Italian) Vinranke (Norwegian) Vid (Spanish) Vin (Swedish)
EU INCI name[2]	*Vitis vinifera*
CTFA INCI name[3]	Grape (*Vitis vinifera*) extract Grape (*Vitis vinifera*) leaf extract Grape (*Vitis vinifera*) seed oil

CAS number	84929-27-1 (extract) 8024-22-4 (seed oil) 85594-37-2 (seed oil)
EINECS number	284-511-6 (extract) 287-896-9 (seed oil)
Parts used	Fruits, leaves, seeds

Important constituents including active principles[13]

Fruits:
- Polyphenols:
  (Flavones: quercetin (traces) and quercitrin, quercetin-, kaempferol- and myricetin-3-monoglucoside, quercetin-glucuronoside, astilbin, engeletin
  Catechins: catechin, epicatechin, gallocatechin, epicatechingallate
  Anthocyanins: delphinidin-, petunidin-, malvidin- (41.2%)[13], cyanidin-, and peonidin-3-monoglucosides
  Procyanidins: procyanidin B_1, B_2, B_3, B_4, B_5, B_7, B_8)
- α-Hydroxyacids (tartaric, citric and malic acids)
- Esters (cont. cinnamic and tartaric acids)
- Aldehydes (vanillin, protocatechuic, cinnamic and coniferyl aldehydes)
- Vitamins (C, B group, PP)

- Carotene
- Sugars (fructose, glucose)
- Polysaccharides (cont. galactose, mannose, arabinose, rhamnose, galacturonic acid)
- Proteins
- Volatile constituents
- Waxes
- Pectin

Seeds:
- Procyanidins (procyanidin B_1, B_2, B_3, B_4, B_5, B_7, B_8)
- Proteins (7-10%)[13] (cont. arginine, cystine, leucine (11.4%)[13], valine, phenylalanine)
- Triglycerides (6-20%)[13] (cont. palmitic, stearic, oleic (37%)[13] and linoleic (55%)13. acids)
- Unsaponifiables (0,5-1%)[11] (phytosterols: b-sitosterol)
- Phospholipids (phosphatidylserine, phosphatidylinositol, lecithin, cephalin, cerebrosides, phosphatidic acid)
- Vitamin E

Leaves:
- Polyphenols:
  (Anthocyanins
  Catechins: catechin, epicatechin, gallocatechin, epicatechin-3-O-gallate)
  Ellagitannins: brevilagin-1, vitilagin and isovitilagin
  Flavones: traces of quercitrin, quercetin, kaempferol, rutin, iso-quercitrin and luteolin)
- Organic acids (tartaric, malic, oxalic, fumaric, succinic, citric and glyceric acids)
- Phenol acids (o- and p-hydroxybenzoic, protocatechuic, gallic, vanillic, syringic and ellargic acids)
- Esters (cont. cinnamic acids and tartaric acid)
- Vitamins (C, PP, B group, folic acid)
- Carotenoids
- Volatile constituents
- Waxes
- Proteins
- Mineral salts (5-7%)[12]

Preparation

1) Extract from fruits
2)[5] "Grape leaf extract"
3)[4] "Grape seed oil"

Manufacturing process

1) Extraction of the leaves with propylene glycol solution
2) Expression of seeds

Examples of specifications

1)[5] pH: 5.0-6.0
   Specific gravity at 20°C: 1.020-1.060
   Heavy metals: not more than 20 ppm
   Arsenic: not more than 2 ppm
   Residue on evaporation: 0.40- 0.70 w/v%

2)[4] Specific gravity at 20°C: 0.917- 0.925
Refractive index at 20°C: 1.475- 1.478
Acid value: not more than 0.5
Saponification value: 187-200
Iodine value: 135-150
Heavy metals: not more 20 ppm
Arsenic: not more than 2 ppm

Intended cosmetic effects and used concentration in cosmetic products

(Fruits)
Dyeing (anthocyanins), protectant, moisturising

(Seeds)
Emollient, protectant, anti-ageing

(Leaves)
Tonic, astringent and refreshing (tannins), anti-ageing

Up to 15% in lotions, creams, gels for ageing skin and hair products

Other possible effects

(Polyphenols)
Free radical scavenger, microcirculation protectant, anti-irritant, antioxidant

(Unsaponifiables)
Granulation promoting agent

Main toxicological data[14, 15]

(Leaf extract)
Primary skin irritation: non-irritant
Acute eye irritation: non-irritant

Databases used

CA Search 1967-98, Medline 1966-98, Embase 1974-98, Ref. Tox. Eff. Chem. Sub., Toxline; Toxbio; Toxcas

Keywords

Vitis vinifera, grape

Evaluation and remarks

Cat. A (fruit extract; leaf extract; seed oil)
No toxicity apparently reported.

General references

1. Index Kewensis, Clarendon Press
2. European Commission Decision 96/335/EC of 8 May 1996, Official Journal of the European Community No. L132 of 1 June 1996
3. International Cosmetic Ingredient Dictionary 6th ed., CTFA, 1995
4. Comprehensive Licensing Standards of Cosmetics by Category, Yakuji Nippo Ltd., *1*, 112, 1986
5. Comprehensive Licensing Standards of Cosmetics by Category, Yakuji Nippo Ltd., *5*, 221, 1990
6. Council of Europe, Flavouring substances and natural sources of flavourings 3rd ed. Maisonneuve, (485 N 1), 1981
7. Fenaroli G., Sostanze Aromatiche Naturali, Hoepli, 978-979, 1963
8. Grieve M., A modern herbal, Barnes & Noble Books, 832, 1996

9. The Japanese Cosmetic Ingredients Codex, ed. Yakuji Nippo Ltd., 336 - 337, 1993

10. Leung A.Y., Foster S, Encyclopedia of Common Natural Ingredients, Wiley & Son Publ., 288-289, 1996

11. Proserpio G., Martelli A., Patri G.F., Elementi di fitocosmesi, Sepem, 2, 792, 842, 1983

12. Van Hellemont J., Compendium de Phytotherapie, APB, 430-431, 1986

Specific references

13. Bombardelli E., Morazzoni P., Vitis vinifera L., Fitoterapia, 66, 4, 291-317, 1995

14. Indena, Product Specification

15. Indena's reports

Members of the Committee of Experts on Cosmetic Products
Membres du Comité d'experts sur les produits cosmétiques

Consultants

Prof. Robert ANTON
Université Louis Pasteur Faculté de Pharmacie
Laboratoire de Pharmacognosie
74, route du Rhin
F-67401 Illkirch cedex

Dr Gianfranco PATRI
INDENA
Via Ortles 12
I-20139 Milano

Prof. Vittorio SILANO
Direttore Generale
Italian Medicines Evaluation and Pharmacovigilance Department
Viale Civilta Romana 7
I-00144 Roma

Austria/Autriche

HR Mag. pharm Dieter JENEWEIN
Head of the Federal Institute for Food Control
Technikerstrasse 70
A-6020 Innsbruck

Dr Aleksander ZILBERSZAC
Federal Chancellery, VI/B/2
Radetzkystraße 2
A-1030 Wien

Dr Aysen HABISON
Federal Institute for Foodstuffs Examination and Research
Head of Dept for the control of cosmetics
Bundesanstalt für Lebensmitteluntersuchung-u-forschung
Kinderspitalgasse 15
A-1090 Wien

Belgium/Belgique

Mr. Jean Marie FEROUMONT
Inspecteur Sanitaire, Inspection Générale des Denrées Alimentaires, Administration de la protection
de la santé, Ministère des Affaires sociales, de la santé publique et de l'environnement
CAE Quartier Esplanade 11.03
Boulevard Pachéco 19, boîte 5
B-1010 Bruxelles

Dr Luc VAN DER MAREN
Expert auprès du Ministère de la Santé Publique Belge
L'OREAL BELGILUX
Rue du Peuplier, 12
B-1000 Bruxelles

Dr. Ph. Marie-Odette MASSE
Chef de travaux agrégé / Chef de Programme – Produits Cosmétiques
Institut Scientifique de Santé Publique – Louis Pasteur
14 rue J. Wytsman
B-1050 Bruxelles

Denmark/Danemark

Mrs Lisbet OLGAARD
Head of Section - Danish Environmental Protection Agency
Strandgade 29
DK-1401 Copenhagen K

Finland/Finlande

Dr Eeva-Liisa SAINIO
Senior Researcher
Consumer Agency
Haapaniemenkatu 4
FIN-00530 Helsinki

France

Mme Catherine CHOMA
Direction Générale de la Santé
Sous-direction de la politique des produits de santé
Bureau des dispositifs médicaux et autres produits de santé (SD3B)
8, Avenue de Ségur
F-75007 Paris

Mme Nathalie CLEMENT
Ministère de l'Industrie – DGSI/SERBCO
3-5 rue Barbet de Jouy
F-75353 Paris 07

Mme Eve-Marie BONNEAU
Chef de la Division Parfums-Cosmétiques-Chimie fine
Secrétariat d'Etat à l'Industrie
Le Bervil - DIGITIP 2 / SIM
12 rue Villiot
F-75572 Paris CEDEX 12

Mme Christiane D'AGATA
Chef du département "Produits cosmétiques"
Agence française de sécurité sanitaire des produits de santé
143-145, boulevard Anatole France
F-93286 Saint Denis

Germany/Allemagne

Dr Regina SCHUMANN
Scientific Co-worker
Bundesinstitut für gesundheitlichen Verbraucherschutz und Veterinärmedizin
Thielallee 88-92, Postfach 33 00 13
D-14195 Berlin

Italy/Italie

Dott.ssa Colomba IACONTINO
Dirigente di II° livello
Ministero della Sanità
Servizio per i Rapporti Internazionali e le Politice Comunitarie
I-00144 Roma EUR

Netherlands/Pays-Bas

Dr Henk ROELFZEMA
Senior Policy Officer
Ministerie VWS/GZB/C&O
Parnassusplein 5 - 2511 VX Den Haag
Postbus 20350
NL-2500 EJ Den Haag

Dr Jan Willem WEIJLAND
Inspectie Waren & Veterinuire Zaken
PO BOX 16108
NL-2500 BC Den Haag

Dr Peter C. BRAGT, Eur. R. Tox.
Senior Officer of Public Health
Inspectorate for Health Protection, Commodities and Veterainary Public Health
Ministry of Health Welfare and Sports
PO BOX 16108
NL-2500 BC Den Haag

Norway/Norvège

Dr Hans Jørgen TALBERG
Adviser – Statens Naeringsmiddeltilsyn (SNT)
Norwegian Food Control Authority - Dept of Food Law and International Affairs
Box 8187 - Ullevålsveien 76
N-0034 Oslo

Portugal

Mme Ana Sofia AMARAL
Expert sur les produits cosmétiques
Instituto Nacional da Farmácia e do Medicamento (INFARMED)
Ministério da Saúde
Parque de Saude de Lisboa
Av. do Brasil, 53
P-1749-004 Lisboa

Mme Maria Amélia JUDICE
Expert sur les produits cosmétiques
Instituto Nacional da Farmácia e do Medicamento (INFARMED)
Ministério da Saúde
Parque de Saude de Lisboa
Av. do Brasil, 53
P-1749-004 Lisboa

Spain/Espagne

Mme María Dolores GRANADOS TEJERO
Chef de Section - Produits Cosmétiques
Direction Générale de la Pharmacie et des Produits Sanitaires
Ministère de la Santé et de la Consommation
Paseo del Prado 18-20
E-28014 Madrid

Sweden/Suède

Ms Anita Finne GRAHNEN
Head of Cosmetic Control
Medical Products Agency
Box 26
S-75103 Uppsala

Mrs Inger NASMAN
Director of Operations
Medical Products Agency
PO Box 26
S-75103 Uppsala

Mrs Kerstin ERNI
Medical Products Agency
Läkemedelsverket, Box 26
S-75103 Uppsala

Switzerland/Suisse

Mme Anna-Barbara WIESMANN
Head of Service of Cosmetics
Federal Office of Public Health
Division of Food Science, Service of Cosmetics
P.O.B
CH-3003 Berne

United Kingdom/Royaume-Uni

Mr David Ratcliffe
Policy Advisor
Consumer Safety Unit
Department of Trade & Industry
Room 432 -1 Victoria Street
GB-London SW1H 0ET

Mr Andrew Lunnon
Consumer Safety Unit
Department of Trade & Industry
Room 4.E.2.
1 Victoria Street
GB-London SW1H 0ET

Secretariat/Secrétariat

Mr Angel RUIZ DE VALBUENA, MD
Administrative Officer/Administrateur
Partial Agreement Department in the Social and Public Health Field
Service de l'Accord partiel dans le domaine social et de la santé publique
Conseil de l'Europe
F-67075 Strasbourg Cedex

Sales agents for publications of the Council of Europe
Agents de vente des publications du Conseil de l'Europe

AUSTRALIA/AUSTRALIE
Hunter Publications, 58A, Gipps Street
AUS-3066 COLLINGWOOD, Victoria
Tel.: (61) 3 9417 5361
Fax: (61) 3 9419 7154
E-mail: Sales@hunter-pubs.com.au
http://www.hunter-pubs.com.au

AUSTRIA/AUTRICHE
Gerold und Co., Weihburggasse 26
A-1010 WIEN
Tel.: (43) 1 533 5014
Fax: (43) 1 533 5014 18
E-mail: buch@gerold.telecom.at
http://www.gerold.at

BELGIUM/BELGIQUE
La Librairie européenne SA
50, avenue A. Jonnart
B-1200 BRUXELLES 20
Tel.: (32) 2 734 0281
Fax: (32) 2 735 0860
E-mail: info@libeurop.be
http://www.libeurop.be

Jean de Lannoy
202, avenue du Roi
B-1190 BRUXELLES
Tel.: (32) 2 538 4308
Fax: (32) 2 538 0841
E-mail: jean.de.lannoy@euronet.be
http://www.jean-de-lannoy.be

CANADA
Renouf Publishing Company Limited
5369 Chemin Canotek Road
CDN-OTTAWA, Ontario, K1J 9J3
Tel.: (1) 613 745 2665
Fax: (1) 613 745 7660
E-mail: order.dept@renoufbooks.com
http://www.renoufbooks.com

CZECH REPUBLIC/
RÉPUBLIQUE TCHÈQUE
USIS, Publication Service
Havelkova 22
CZ-130 00 PRAHA 3
Tel.: (420) 2 210 02 111
Fax: (420) 2 242 21 1484
E-mail: posta@uvis.cz
http://www.usiscr.cz/

DENMARK/DANEMARK
Swets Blackwell A/S
Jagtvej 169 B, 2 Sal
DK-2100 KOBENHAVN O
Tel.: (45) 39 15 79 15
Fax: (45) 39 15 79 10
E-mail: info@dk.swetsblackwell.com

FINLAND/FINLANDE
Akateeminen Kirjakauppa
Keskuskatu 1, PO Box 218
FIN-00381 HELSINKI
Tel.: (358) 9 121 41
Fax: (358) 9 121 4450
E-mail: akatilaus@stockmann.fi
http://www.akatilaus.akateeminen.com

FRANCE
La Documentation française
124 rue H. Barbusse
93308 Aubervilliers Cedex
Tel.: (33) 01 40 15 70 00
Fax: (33) 01 40 15 68 00
E-mail: commandes.vel@ladocfrancaise.gouv.fr
http://www.ladocfrancaise.gouv.fr

GERMANY/ALLEMAGNE
UNO Verlag
Am Hofgarten 10
D-53113 BONN
Tel.: (49) 2 28 94 90 20
Fax: (49) 2 28 94 90 222
E-mail: unoverlag@aol.com
http://www.uno-verlag.de

GREECE/GRÈCE
Librairie Kauffmann
Mavrokordatou 9
GR-ATHINAI 106 78
Tel.: (30) 1 38 29 283
Fax: (30) 1 38 33 967

HUNGARY/HONGRIE
Euro Info Service
Hungexpo Europa Kozpont ter 1
H-1101 BUDAPEST
Tel.: (361) 264 8270
Fax: (361) 264 8271
E-mail: euroinfo@euroinfo.hu
http://www.euroinfo.hu

ITALY/ITALIE
Libreria Commissionaria Sansoni
Via Duca di Calabria 1/1, CP 552
I-50125 FIRENZE
Tel.: (39) 556 4831
Fax: (39) 556 41257
E-mail: licosa@licosa.com
http://www.licosa.com

NETHERLANDS/PAYS-BAS
De Lindeboom Internationale Publikaties
PO Box 202, MA de Ruyterstraat 20 A
NL-7480 AE HAAKSBERGEN
Tel.: (31) 53 574 0004
Fax: (31) 53 572 9296
E-mail: lindeboo@worldonline.nl
http://home-1-worldonline.nl/~lindeboo/

NORWAY/NORVÈGE
Akademika, A/S Universitetsbokhandel
PO Box 84, Blindern
N-0314 OSLO
Tel.: (47) 22 85 30 30
Fax: (47) 23 12 24 20

POLAND/POLOGNE
Głowna Księgarnia Naukowa
im. B. Prusa
Krakowskie Przedmiescie 7
PL-00-068 WARSZAWA
Tel.: (48) 29 22 66
Fax: (48) 22 26 64 49
E-mail: inter@internews.com.pl
http://www.internews.com.pl

PORTUGAL
Livraria Portugal
Rua do Carmo, 70
P-1200 LISBOA
Tel.: (351) 13 47 49 82
Fax: (351) 13 47 02 64
E-mail: liv.portugal@mail.telepac.pt

SPAIN/ESPAGNE
Mundi-Prensa Libros SA
Castelló 37
E-28001 MADRID
Tel.: (34) 914 36 37 00
Fax: (34) 915 75 39 98
E-mail: libreria@mundiprensa.es
http://www.mundiprensa.com

SWITZERLAND/SUISSE
BERSY
Route de Monteiller
CH-1965 SAVIESE
Tel.: (41) 27 395 53 33
Fax: (41) 27 395 53 34
E-mail: jprausis@netplus.ch

Adeco – Van Diermen
Chemin du Lacuez 41
CH-1807 BLONAY
Tel.: (41) 21 943 26 73
Fax: (41) 21 943 36 06
E-mail: mvandier@worldcom.ch

UNITED KINGDOM/ROYAUME-UNI
TSO (formerly HMSO)
51 Nine Elms Lane
GB-LONDON SW8 5DR
Tel.: (44) 207 873 8372
Fax: (44) 207 873 8200
E-mail: customer.services@theso.co.uk
http://www.the-stationery-office.co.uk
http://www.itsofficial.net

UNITED STATES and CANADA/
ÉTATS-UNIS et CANADA
Manhattan Publishing Company
468 Albany Post Road, PO Box 850
CROTON-ON-HUDSON,
NY 10520, USA
Tel.: (1) 914 271 5194
Fax: (1) 914 271 5856
E-mail: Info@manhattanpublishing.com
http://www.manhattanpublishing.com

STRASBOURG
Librairie Kléber
Palais de l'Europe
F-67075 STRASBOURG Cedex
Fax: (33) 03 88 52 91 21

Council of Europe Publishing/Editions du Conseil de l'Europe
F-67075 Strasbourg Cedex
Tel.: (33) 03 88 41 25 81 – Fax: (33) 03 88 41 39 10
E-mail: publishing@coe.int – Web site: http://book.coe.int